From an educational perspective this text provides <barcode> I0048983
to construct during professional training alongside
with the various clinical skills and competencies expected of a quality
health professional. What this text clearly portrays is that the way you
communicate and conduct yourself with your patients and the public at
large is a core value that must never be compromised.

> Prof. David Byfield
> Head of Clinical Services, Welsh Institute of Chiropractic
> University of South Wales, UK

Dr. Kinsinger has written a must-study primer for anyone entering
or currently practicing in a healthcare profession. Learn from one of
the best with this well-compiled book, full of important information
for those wanting to establish strength-based relationships with their
patients and colleagues.

> Michal A. Mestan, DC, EdD
> President, Northeast College of Health Sciences, NY

This text provides the clinician with insight and guidance to navigate
the turbulent health care environment. Within the pages that follow
are skills and abilities that strengthen one's professional foundation;
"survival skills" that support and bolster the professionalism intrinsic
to health care.

> Nancy Kirsch, PT, DPT, PhD, FAPTA,
> Professor, Doctor of Physical Therapy Program,
> Rutgers University, NJ

This book is a welcome addition to the body of information related to the
ethics of healthcare. It addresses some of the fundamental issues that
healthcare practitioners grapple with and lays out the issues in a clear,

thoughtful and practical presentation that makes it an ideal text for use in educating students intending to become healthcare professionals.

Professor Christina Cunliffe, PhD, DC, CBiol, FRSB, FCC (Paeds), FMCA

Principal, McTimoney College of Chiropractic, UK

Dr. Kinsinger, a practitioner and educator with a long and strong history of teaching professional ethics, has produced a concise and useful guidebook for practitioners. The book is well laid-out, clearly stated and includes a number of case examples (called "You be the Judge") which are very useful in applying the book's concepts. An excellent text for guiding professional behavior, especially in a chiropractic context.

Brian McAulay, DC, PhD

Vice President of Academic Affairs, Logan University, MO

This text is a vital resource for chiropractic educational programs. I highly recommend it as a core reference for ethics and professional courses. Each chapter includes a "You Be the Judge section" with verdicts. These summaries provide students and educators an opportunity to reflect and discuss ethical challenges that occur in practice in an experiential learning environment.

Lynn B. Pownall, DC, DACNB, CHSE

Clinical Associate Professor, School of Health Professions, Chiropractic Program, D'Youville University, NY

Demonstrating leadership is the most crucial element missing in the profession and should be a requirement within all chiropractic program curricula and continuing education licensing requirements.

Michael A. Ciolfi, DC, MBA, DBA

Dean, College of Health Sciences, University of Bridgeport, CT

Principles of Professionalism in Health Care is a well-crafted manuscript and an accurate reflection of what Dr. Kinsinger has dedicated much of his life to understand and teach: ethics and professionalism. While it is highly intellectual, it is neither pretentious nor ponderous. This easy-to-read book is the preferred text of professionalism in healthcare.

> *William E. Morgan, DC, DAAPM, FICC, FIM, FPAC, LLD (hc)*
> *President Parker University, TX*

Principles of Professionalism in Health Care pulls no punches helping the reader sort through contrasting concepts such as the difference between privacy and confidentiality, ethics versus morals and the challenge of moral relativism in our times. It presents actual cases to judge at the end of each chapter. This is a wonderful book for learners and seasoned practitioners alike to return to often, along their own professionalism journey.

> *Michael Kaufmann, MD, FCFP, FASAM, FISAM, ABAM dip*
> *Founding Director of the Physician Health Program,*
> *Ontario Medical Association*

Whether a health professional is looking for initial education on key ethical concepts or a refresher about an under-appreciated aspect of health professional curricula, Stuart Kinsinger's whirlwind tour of ethics and professionalism in health care provides remarkably applicable content. The practical guidance about complex ethical issues in this manuscript is delivered in approachable terms with clever tips and activities that are certain to help readers retain what they have learned. Health professionals and regulatory bodies alike would benefit from reading Dr. Kinsinger's work.

> *Mark Staz, MA, Federation of State Medical Boards, USA*

Principles of Professionalism in Health Care provides an excellent reference text for the development of the professional learner into the profession. Each chapter has been purposely constructed with theory supported by experiential learning with the "Searches and Scenarios" and "You be the Judge" at the conclusion.

Assoc Prof Navine Haworth
Academic Dean
Australian Chiropractic College

❧

Principles of Professionalism
in Health Care

❧

ॐ

Principles
of
Professionalism
in
Health Care

A GUIDE TO BUILDING
RELATIONSHIPS OF TRUST

F. Stuart Kinsinger

ॐ

foreword by Richard Cruess, MD, CC,
and Sylvia Cruess, MD, OC

Library and Archives Canada Cataloguing in Publication Data
Kinsinger, F. Stuart, 1952–
        Principles of professionalism in health care : a guide to building relationships of trust / Stuart Kinsinger.
Includes bibliographical references.

ISBN 978-0-9781421-1-7 (print edition)
ISBN 978-0-9781421-2-4 (epub)

1. Health care providers – Professional ethics. 2. Chiropractors – Professional ethics. 3. Physical therapists – Professional ethics. 4. Masseurs – Professional ethics. 5. Naturopaths – Professional ethics. 6. Acupuncturists – Professional ethics. I. Title.
RZ236.5.K55 2022   174.2'95534   C2022-904110-5
Revised and expanded edition of *Principles of Professionalism for Manual Therapists: A Guide to Building Relationships of Trust*, ISBN 0-9781421-0-1, published 2006, reprinted 2012.

Published by:
Dr. F. Stuart Kinsinger
www.DrKinsinger.com
stuart@DrKinsinger.com

Design: Counterpunch Inc. / Linda Gustafson

*I am grateful for having had the privilege to pursue two careers:
managing patients' musculoskeletal concerns, and translating
professionalism principles to learners. Foundational to this
has been the "home team" without whose love, support, and blessing,
such privilege would not have been realized.*

*This book is dedicated to my wife, Laurel,
daughter, Melissa, and son, Ted, with thanks.*

Contents

Foreword to the First Edition: Professionalism versus Professionalization

Ian D. Coulter Ph.D.

Health consultant, Rand, Santa Monica, California
Professor, School of Dentistry, University of California, Los Angeles
Professor, Southern California University of Health Sciences

The approach to professions within sociology and society has followed an interesting trajectory. At one time within society the professions were seen as the pinnacle of achievement for groups within certain occupations to establish their credibility. The three most prestigious professions – medicine, the law and the priesthood – were held up as exemplars of achievement and ones that other social groups could emulate. Beginning around the 1960s we have seen an open revolt against medicine including such groups as the feminist movement and the consumer movement. Jokes about lawyers are now abundant: "How does one know when a lawyer is lying? When you see his/her lips move." Such jokes reflect a deep dissatisfaction with what lawyers, if not the laws themselves, have become. The priesthood sees itself under attack in virtually all countries because of sexual abuse of minors. So all three of these once proud and respected professions finds themselves under social attack so much so that the word "professional" has almost become a negative term.

Within sociology the work has gone from seeing professions as having definable characteristics, especially acting in the public interest and always putting the public interest ahead of the selfinterest of the members of the professions, to seeing such groups as medicine as examples of dominance. Here professions are seen as political organizations whose primary interest is advancing their own agendas. So the work has gone from seeing the groups as the helping professions to seeing them as groups helping themselves to the detriment of the public.

This state of affairs would have been almost inconceivable in the 1950s and raises the question of what happened to the professions. It also poses a significant challenge for those groups who are aspiring to become professions in their own right and for works such as this, which lay out the requirements for a profession and a road map for how they might be achieved. It raises the question: "Is professionalism worth pursuing?"

Part of the problem is that many groups forgot that professionalism is a process, not a destination. While it is important to recognize that the process involves achieving certain characteristics (such as a code of ethics), these structural features are not the final achievement. We should talk about professionalization as a process, not professionalism as finished work.

The second part of the problem is that professionalism is invariably about social power. In fact professions are given incredible power by the state. They can control who joins the profession, they can control the whole process of regulation of the members of the profession, they can often remove someone from the profession and they can discipline non-members for practicing within the scope of practice reserved for the profession. They may also be given the power to define a whole area of activity like health and be the defining body for wide areas of social policy. In return for this extraordinary power, professions were obligated to act in the public interest. It is the failure to do this while at the same time publicly claiming to do so that has got professions into trouble. The claim has been so blatantly false that the public has lost faith with the professions. With the lost of faith came the loss of respect.

The challenge therefore is how to return professions back to the process of professionalization. This process might be partly achieved through such efforts as contained in this work: education. The principles of professionalization are clearly noble and worthy of being embraced. But they must be re-taught, re-emphasized with each new generation and, more important, constantly modeled by those in practice. Professionalization must be as much caught as taught. This work provides an important starting point but it is only that. It deals with the rhetoric of professionalization, but it is behavior that deals with the reality. Ultimately professionalization is about acting professionally. It takes a long time to learn to be professional and it takes a lifetime to practice it. It takes no more than a few minutes to destroy it. In the words of Shakespeare:

"Mine honour is my life, both grow in one;
 Take honour from me and my life is done."
   Richard II, Shakespeare

Foreword to the Second Edition

Richard Cruess, MD, CC, Dean Emeritus and Professor Emeritus of Surgery and Health Sciences Education; McGill University
Sylvia Cruess, MD, OC, Professor Emerita of Medicine and Health Sciences Education; McGill University

Robert Merton's introduction to a work that was the first study of the sociology of medical education provides an oft quoted statement that is appropriate as an entrée into this Foreword. He wrote that it is the task of professional education to *"transmit the culture of medicine and to shape the novice into an effective practitioner of medicine, to give him the best available knowledge and skills, and to provide him with a professional identity so that he comes to think, act, and feel like a physician."*[1] We have come to understand that for all professions, while challenging, it is relatively easy to determine and communicate knowledge and skills. However, in the increasingly interconnected and complex world in which professionals must function, it is truly challenging to ensure that practitioners think act, and feel like the professional that the public needs, desires and, indeed, expects.[2,3] In part the difficulty arises because the educational institutions and regulatory bodies that are mandated to produce professionals have come to understand the necessity for preparing practitioners so that they may function not only in today's world, but in a future whose external conditions will be substantially different from today. Thus, a primary objective of professional education is to ensure that graduates and practitioners are prepared for change and can adapt to ever-changing conditions.

While it is clear that change will occur, a challenge that is perhaps more daunting and difficult is how we determine what in our present and past must be preserved in the thoughts, beliefs, and actions of these individuals who must change. Only in this way can we be true to the history of service to society that has long been an aspirational goal of the professions.[2,3]

The concept of professionalism and its role in the education and maintenance of competence of future professionals is foundational to addressing the issue. There are several reasons for this. The historical values of the professional are encompassed within the meaning of the word professional and their manifestation is an ongoing indication of the professionalism of those who espouse it.[4] Dr. Kinsinger outlines these characteristics in several places in this excellent book. Throughout the ages these values were not taught explicitly in the curriculum of professional schools.[5] It was assumed that learners would come to understand and exhibit them implicitly by modelling their behaviour on that of instructors whom they admired and respected. It has been amply demonstrated that this informal approach, by itself is no longer sufficient. Therefore in an attempt to ensure that all learners at least understood what was expected of them by the professional community that they were attempting to join,[6] most professional schools began to teach professionalism explicitly.[5] This required developing definitions which had generally been absent and creating a cognitive base that could be communicated, along with other knowledge and skills[7] In addition, methods of assessing professional behaviours in a fair and psychometrically sound fashion were developed.[8] This reinforced the importance of definitions and lists of attributes. If something is to be taught and assessed effectively, it must be defined and both instructors and learners must understand the definition and list of attributes.

The second reason for the role of professionalism in the world of the professions is that, as institutions began explicitly teaching professionalism, an awareness gradually developed that knowledge of professionalism alone was insufficient.[9] The belief systems and attributes of the profession must become an integral part of the identity of the practitioner. The educational objective should therefore be to support individuals as they develop a professional identity, with the attributes of the professional and professionalism serving as the basis of that identity.[10] Thus, even if professional identity becomes the educational objective, professionalism still must be taught as its basis.[11] Finally, and not often articulated, professionalism as a word is inherently important because it includes those beliefs and value systems that society has come to expect of those serving it in the professions. As is outlined in this wonderful book, the professions and professionalism serve as the basis of the social contract between medicine and society.[4,12] The professions are granted a privileged position in society and substantial financial and nonfinancial rewards along with considerable autonomy in practice and the privilege of self-regulation. In return they are expected to ensure the competence of their fellow practitioners, demonstrate morality and integrity in all of their professional and nonprofessional activities and consistently place their personal interest and the interest of their profession above that of their patients, clients, and society. As this is a social contract in which society is actually granting status to the professions, the failure of individual practitioners or of the professions as a whole to meet societal expectations will result in society changing the nature of the social contract, generally by altering or withdrawing privileges from the professions.[12] As is little understood, the failure of society to meet the legitimate expectations of the professions also has unforeseen and generally unwanted consequences. The professions generally change their behaviour having lost the trust in society that is so essential to the maintenance of the contract.[12] This book properly emphasizes this risk.

A final note, we live in a world where much of the scholarly work on professions and professionalism has been carried out in the Anglo-American world.[2,3] For many years the understanding that resulted was considered to be not only a benchmark but also relatively universal and unchanging. As we have embraced an understanding of the world as a global family it has become obvious that professionalism is a social construct that is neither immutable or universal. It changes as societal needs and expectations change in a world where healthcare and legal structures are in constant flux. Even the Anglo-American concept of professionalism has altered considerably in the past few decades.[13] Furthermore the concept of professionalism exists in other nations, cultures and religious settings and there are substantial differences between the Anglo-American concept and the rest of the world.[12] This has greatly altered our understanding of the professions and professionalism; also reflected in this text.

In closing it seems worthwhile to emphasize how important professionalism is to the individual professional and to their professional organizations. Professional status is hugely beneficial to the individual practitioner, leading to both status and financial and nonfinancial rewards. However, it must be stressed that if this were the only reason for the existence of the privileged position of the professions, it is doubtful that it would represent sufficient justification for their existence. It is however, a benefit to society being the basis for the essential "trusting relationship" described by the author. William Sullivan, a social scientist and philosopher has provided a quote that will close this Foreword:

"Neither economic incentives, nor technology, nor administrative control has proved an effective surrogate for the commitment to integrity invoked in the ideal of professionalism".[4]

Principles of Professionalism in Health Care: a Guide to Building Relationships of Trust is a most welcome addition to the tools available to those responsible for the formation of practitioners within the healthcare system and for the organizations whose mandate is to ensure that the professions conduct themselves in a way that merits societal trust. It is a powerful combination of theory, that allows us to understand the task at hand, and practical guides for its implementation. The section entitled "You be the judge" is particularly useful as it highlights the points of tension inherent in practice and allows learners to reflect on these issues in a safe environment.

As is so true of most of the works which advance our knowledge of professionalism, this important book has the potential to have a positive impact on healthcare with beneficial results to both society and individual patients.

Note to reader: This Foreword represents the last collaboration between the author and his beloved wife and partner of 62 years, Sylvia Cruess. She was an equal participant in all of our joint contributions and in the conception of this final work, but sadly passed away before it was completed. It is dedicated to her memory with love and gratitude.

REFERENCES

1. Merton, R.K., Reader, L.G., Kendall, P.L. (eds.), *The student physician: introductory studies in the sociology of medical education.* (Cambridge MA: Harvard University Press, 1957).
2. Starr, P., *The Social Transformation of American Medicine* (New York: Basic Books, 2nd edition and Epilogue, 2016).

3. Krause, E., *Death of the Guilds: Professions, States and the Advance of Capitalism, 1930 to the Present,* (New Haven: Yale University Press, 1996).

4. Sullivan, W., *Work and Integrity: The Crisis and Promise of Professionalism in North America* (New York: Harper Collins, 2nd edition, 2005).

5. Cruess, S.R., Cruess, R.L., *Professionalism must be taught* (BJM, 1997) 315: 1674–1677.

6. Cruess, R.L., Cruess, S.R., Steinert, Y., "Medicine as a community of practice: implications for medical education" (2018) *Academic Medicine* 92: 185–195.

7. Cruess, R., Cruess, S., "Teaching Professionalism: general principles" (2006) *Medical Teacher* 28 205–208.

8. Wilkinson, T. J., Wade, W. B., Knock, L.D., "A blueprint to assess professionalism: results of a systematic review" (2009) *Academic Medicine* 84: 551-55898.

9. Cooke, M., Irby, D.M., O'Brien, C., *Educating physicians: a call for reform of medical school and residency* (San Francisco: Jossey-Bass, 2010).

10. Cruess, R.L., Cruess, S.R., Boudreau, D.B., Snell, L., Steinert, Y., "Reframing medical education to support the development of professional identity formation." (2014) *Academic Medicine* 89:1446-1451

11. Cruess, R.L., Cruess, S.R., Steinert, Y. (eds.), *Teaching medical professionalism: supporting the development of a professional identity* (Cambridge University Press, 2nd edition, 2016)

12. Cruess, R.L., Cruess, S.R., "Expectations and obligations: professionalism and medicine's social contract with society" (2008) *Perspectives in Biology and Medicine* 51: 579-598

13. Hafferty, F.W., Castellani, B., "A sociological framing of medicine's modern-day professionalism movement (2009) *Medical Education* 43: 826-828.

14. Ho, M-J., Yu, K-H., Hirsh, D., Huang, T-S., Yang, P-C., "Does one size fit all? Building a framework for medical professionalism" (2011) *Academic Medicine* 86: 1407-1414.

Preface

"I'm not sure I can define it, but I sure know it when I see it" captures the challenge when contemplating "professionalism." Thankfully the struggle to offer a cogent definition is ameliorated by practitioners who exemplify and fulfil its highest expression in the provision of health care.

Research, regulation and education make up the "foundation triad" that establishes a profession's *raison d'etre*. Unpacking the scholarship illuminates a profession's length, breadth and depth. Translating this to learners is an awesome privilege ... challenges and all.

This text follows *Principles of Professionalism for Manual Therapists (2006)* as a companion volume. It is a scientific, evidence-based exploration of professionalism in all its domains. Each chapter sets out professional ideals and responsibilities and ends with focused activities intended to sharpen the learner's insight.

A "Professionalism Venn Diagram" illustrates the interpersonal dynamic of the health care encounter; the interaction between two parties; one in the position of authority and the other in need of a healing touch.

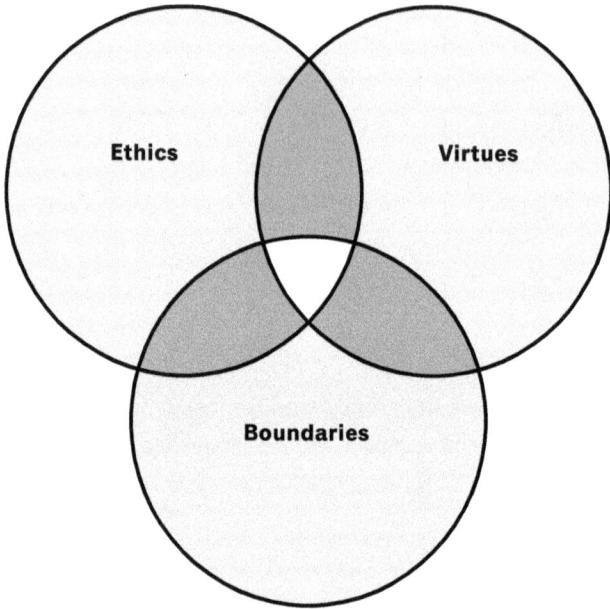

Each circle holds specific and strategic tenets and values. It's in the overlap that a critical mass of our professional identity emerges. Professional duties and responsibilities inspire us to hold ourselves and each other to the highest standards. As under the Social Contract, society demands we do our part, and do it well.

The rewards are inestimable. No practitioner retires from an active practice caring for patients and wonders if their life's work made a difference in the lives of others. Embrace the calling. Marvel in the privilege.

F.S. Kinsinger, DC, MA

ᛦ

Principles of Professionalism
in Health Care

ᛦ

What do Professionals Profess?

To profess. The definition from Oxford: "to claim that something is true or correct" and more broadly "stating openly what you claim."

Similarly, *profession* is uncomplicated. Oxford: "the occupation which one professes to be skilled in and to follow." This expands to "a vocation in which professed knowledge of an aspect of learning is used in its application to the affairs of others."

Professionals profess to the world expertise predicated on specific ideals that define a profession. Principles, values, ethics and virtues are professed by one holding specialized skills, knowledge and experience, with an unwavering commitment to use this expertise for the benefit of others.

The Professions

Which occupations are called professions? At what point does a craft, skilled task or therapy reach the threshold in meeting the high standards of a profession?

Law, medicine and the clergy were the original professions. Over time other disciplines were accorded the designation. More recently many jurisdictions have legislated and regulated newer groups such as Kinesiology and Traditional Chinese Medicine. All professions have taken the necessary steps to position themselves as professionals worthy of the high standards society requires.

About the Word

The word is used incorrectly by those whose work does not meet the standard of the defining characteristics. For example, the word "professional" is sometimes used to describe a business owner or entrepreneur who passionately pursues a worthy business venture.

While the love of excellence, pursuit of client happiness, and strict adherence to high standards are admirable goals and objectives for anyone engaged in the business world, they do not define a profession.

Society blurs the lines between skills, vocations, occupations and professions. One important observation is that professional work has always been collegial and collaborative rather than entrepreneurial, competitive and profit driven.

Professional athletes are paid to play their sport. But athletes are not professionals in the same way that business owners or entrepreneurs are likewise not professionals. Athletes may exemplify many worthy attributes, but their work does not define the qualities of a profession or professionalism.

Professionalism's Set

The two foundational pillars of every profession are control over a specialized body of knowledge, and a commitment to use this expertise for the good of others.

Professionalism can be expressed in seven distinguishing principles; these collectively forming the *"set"* of professionalism:

1. There exists a defined body of knowledge and skills, with this knowledge built upon rational theories and established fact, and disseminated in scholarly publications and related academic venues.

2. There is a long and formal education process, culminating in qualifications sufficient to meet working standards, with the terms and conditions established by those already engaged in practice.

3. The work and knowledge are controlled and organized by associations largely independent of states and governments.

4. The mandate of these associations is formalized by written documents which include state or jurisdictional laws that govern authority, licensure, continuing education and conduct.

5. Individual members practicing under the authority of these associations remain largely autonomous, so long as they work within prescribed regulations.

6. There is a commitment to serve in one's area of expertise including the relief and prevention of pain and suffering, participating in researching newer and safer practices, serving as an authority in public affairs related to one's domain, and valuing performance and the public's interest above financial reward.

7. Individual members are held to a higher standard of behavior than non-members, ensuring public trust.

Embodied in these seven tenets is one professing to society the promise of being worthy of trust, professing never to use specialized skills for self service and self reward, but always and without exception, to use such expertise for the greater good, benefitting society.

Professionalism's Setting

The *"setting"* of professionalism is found in how the professional's work is positioned. It is the delivery of one's skills that forms the "setting" of professionalism in which the "set" rests.

Public members are readily able to identify attributes they deem as professional. Patients note a practitioner's apparel and appearance, an empathic attitude and communication skills as being important.

Having first defined the "set" comprising the seven defining characteristics of a profession, it is the *"setting"* that facilitates the delivery of the practitioner's skills. While there is scant literature on the "setting," three important and tangible building blocks form the "setting" within which the "set" resides.

1. INTERPERSONAL SKILLS

Well developed interpersonal skills honor every aspect of the healing encounter. While interpersonal skills are neither the defining hallmark nor the distinguishing feature of professionalism, a professional without good "people skills" limits the benefits of care.

Young learners and practitioners realize most of their patients are older than they are. Professionals can readily facilitate communication with patients in their middle and senior years using an honorific: calling them by their title and surname: Mr. So-and-so or Ms. How-do-you-do. Patients in an older demographic were taught this was how one demonstrated respect. Experienced practitioners will tell you older patients prefer to be called by their first name; this after they get to know you.

The ability to communicate with ease and compassion is an essential part of facilitating the healing process. First impressions reign supreme. Presenting oneself in a direct, friendly and caring way provides a nurturing "setting" in which to deliver the goods, the "set."

2. APPEARANCE MATTERS

Health care students come to realize that appearance is important. Patients have an expectation of how a professional should look. Like it or not, we must take care to understand how this expectation fits into work as a provider.

It is unlikely that the last time you visited your doctor, chiropractor, massage or physical therapist she or he was wearing a baseball cap, shorts and flip flops, unless you were competing in an elite event and being treated in the rehab tent.

Baseball caps, toques and ripped jeans may be tolerated in classes, but they are forbidden by dress codes in patient clinics where students work with the public.

Your professors and clinicians tell you that casual wear is not part of how a professional should look. For this reason, appearance does matter. It is subjective and culturally based, but is one reality of professionals being held to a higher standard.

In the first book of its kind back in the 1970s, wardrobe engineer John Molloy, studied how dress and appearance affect our attitudes and reactions. *Dress for Success* was written for younger boomers moving up the corporate and professional ladder, by seeking insight in how images generated from clothing provide a vehicle for financial success.

Though fashion styles change, the advice stands. Overdressing can be just as unhelpful as being dressed too casually. Successful health care professionals tend to follow upper-middle class clothing styles. In order to present a professional appearance be neat, wear clean and pressed clothing and shine your shoes.

Current fashion styles are not helpful in giving guidance on what is least likely to offend. Revealing clothing may be trendy, but should not be worn when treating patients. As professionals we honor the fiduciary covenant in all that we do, including our appearance.

A white-coat clinic jacket always presents a good clinical look and has the additional benefit of giving the patient a visual manifestation of the boundary between practitioner and patient. Practice good hygiene, especially with the face, hair and nails.

3. AN ATTITUDINAL ADJUSTMENT

There is little published evidence on the attitude one brings to the professional – patient clinical encounter. Practice management seminars are available in most disciplines, often as strategy to increase one's income. Attendees are told one of the hallmark features of success is to have a positive attitude and a success oriented, outgoing personality.

Anecdotal evidence for this is strong. This positive attitude can be delivered in multiple ways, but no double blind, randomized control trial needs to be conducted in order to show that patents have greater satisfaction with the clinical encounter when their professional is engaged and gives every appearance of enjoying the opportunity to serve.

Attentive listening, a genuine smile, eye contact, affirming words and a positive attitude are essential components to the "setting' of professionalism.

Hippocrates

"For some patients, though conscious that their condition is perilous, recover their health simply through their contentment with the goodness of the physician."

The Social Contract

The social contract between society and the professions is relatively new compared with the Hippocratic Oath, though both share a promise made to society. A critical mass of the social contract emerged as advances in early health care delivery occurred in the 19th century.

Benefits are reciprocal. The greater good for society is the benefit to patients. Society reciprocates with terms and conditions that enable and facilitate individual practitioners in the provision of care. Clinical expertise is essential in a modern society and the professional's power is to be used beneficently.

Though not written out, the contract is a deal and both parties have obligations to uphold. Professors Richard and Sylvia Cruess's scholarship has greatly helped our understanding of the "deal."

Society has the expectation that health professions provide:
- Competent health care services
- High standards of morals and ethics
- Subordination of practitioners' interests over patients'
- Transparency and accountability.

Professions have the expectation that society provide members:
- A monopoly on the provision of their expertise
- A functional health care system
- Status and financial reward
- Self-regulation.

Both parties' expectations are foundational to the provision of care. Each side has the expectation that the terms will be honored and enforced. Non-compliance is given high priority to ensure the integrity of the deal continues to future generations.

By placing the "Set" in the "Setting" we professes our professionalism as follows.

What Do Professionals Profess?

1. **Uphold the Social Contract:** While the Social Contract concerns itself with how the professions and society interact, individual practitioners have an obligation to know its terms and conditions and uphold them. Our obligations are reciprocated, as society rewards us by providing a system that facilitates the provision of care. For the practitioner, simply putting the patient first is not enough. We must early come to grips with the reality that, as professionals, we are held to higher standards in all aspects of our life and not just in a work setting.

2. **Act as a Moral Agent:** Professionals occupy a position of power, trust and authority. We use this position to advocate for the benefit of our patients, and to influence our communities for good. Moral agency obligates us to use power as change agents in accordance with an objective and keen moral compass.

3. **Practice Ethically:** We advocate for and uphold the well-articulated ethics of care beginning with the foundational tenets of autonomy, beneficence, justice and nonmaleficence. The broader mosaic weaves in the virtues which include empathy, trust, altruism, fortitude, honesty and integrity.

4. **Protect the vulnerable:** Patient care is inherently intimate because of the close interpersonal proximity between the parties. The privilege of touch and the practitioner's responsibility to take the greatest of care with this healing touch enables and facilitates patient outcomes and wellbeing. As under the auspices of the Social Contract's power differential, the health care professional is, always and without exception, responsible for setting and maintaining a healthy and functional boundary. Above all, we do no harm.

5. **Be honest and truthful:** While honesty is a key, non-negotiable virtue there are enormous pressures on practitioners to ensure all aspects of business are unflinchingly honest and accurate, including conflicts of interest being well managed. All documents and clinical records must fully adhere to the truth. Signatures, both written and electronic, must be used carefully and intentionally.

6. **Keep private things confidential:** Patients reveal personal and intimate details of their lives. Why do they bare their souls and bodies? Trust. They trust us to keep private things confidential. Any violation of the trust-bond between doctor and patient harms the patient and besmirches the reputation of the profession.

7. **Communicate empathetically:** Patients demand that we communicate with clarity and empathy. Online, professionals are obligated to manage social media ensuring digital footprints honor and respect the principles of professionalism. Misuse constitutes professional misconduct.

8. **Model optimal health and wellness:** While stress, overwork and burnout are widespread in health care, they are antithetical to the principles of good health. The duty to be self-aware and pursue self-care, actively modeling optimal health and wellness, constitutes part of the individual practitioner's responsibility as under the Social Contract. An unwell practitioner is a risk to patients, the public and the profession.

9. **Maintain clinical competence:** The Social Contract imposes a duty requiring members of a profession to maintain competencies based on evidence-based clinical advancements. This commitment to "life long learning" strengthens the trust bond between patient, practitioner and profession.

10. **Honor and uphold the profession:** Learners embark on a unique professionalization journey. The acquisition of knowledge, skills

and values acculturates a young professional through a complex socialization and knowledge translation process. This is termed Professional Identity Formation. Professional work is a highly esteemed privilege. All practitioners are duty bound to nurture and uphold the honor of their profession in order to be worthy of public trust.

Professors Cruess & Cruess

An online search for "professionalism" produces multiple citations from Professors Richard and Sylvia Cruess. They are the reigning academicians of professionalism scholarship and have used their positions at McGill University to uncover much of the scholarship on professionalism. Since 1970 they have published over 25 peer reviewed papers defining and quantifying how professionalism is embedded in the enterprise of health care. Their contribution to the literature is without equal. Educators and clinicians around the globe honor them with deep appreciation and gratitude.

Scenarios and Searches

a. A succinct definition of the word "professionalism" has proven elusive compared with other terms used in this chapter. Create one using this chapter's content.

b. Reflect on your own professionalization journey. What motivated you to apply to your program? How far back did you foresee your future in health care? Was this felt as a calling?

c. Search for "change agent" and "social change agent." How do you see the art and philosophy of your practice fulfilling this role?

d. Professional dress codes are cultural and contextual. Does your profession publish anything on this? What constitutes unacceptable apparel when treating patients?

You be the judge

A 20 year old female attended to a chiropractor complaining of shoulder pain of three days duration. It was early September and she was preparing to return to university. The chiropractor diagnosed a capsular strain, provided initial treatment, assigned home care and a follow up visit two days on.

A week later the patient's mother called the office and told the chiropractor her daughter ended up in a hospital emergency department one day after the second visit. The patient developed severe shortness of breath and was assessed as having a pulmonary embolism.

The chiropractor reviewed the clinical notes making some edits and additions to the chart, but did not indicate these changes were per the information provided by the mother. The regulator received a complaint alleging clinical deficiency on the part of the chiropractor. The investigation focused on all aspects of the clinical encounter. The practitioner provided both a statement and the clinical notes; all forming key parts of evidence. The investigation found:

    a. The patient's history and examination were thorough;

    b. It is highly unlikely an otherwise healthy 20 year old would suffer an embolic event;

    c. The edits to the chart notes gave the appearance of embellishing or covering up some of the diagnostic workup.

You be the judge? Should the chiropractor be found guilty of clinical misconduct due to an incorrect diagnosis? Does making an addition to a chart note constitute misconduct?

Further Resources & References

Keeping current with scholarly evidence upholds our end of the Social Contract "deal." In this way we nurture the integrity of the profession; one of our professional obligations.

First things first: always start by reading your licensing body's published guidelines and standards of practice *before* expanding your search. They matter most.

CHAPTER 1 WHAT DO PROFESSIONALS PROFESS?

Cruess, R.L., Cruess, S.R., "Professionalism, communities of practice, and medicine's social contract," *Journal of the American Board of Family Medicine*, 2020.

Cruess, S.R., Cruess, R.L., Steinert, Y., "Supporting the development of a professional identity: general principles," *Medical Teacher,* 2019.

Iserson, K.V., "Talking about professionalism through the lens of professional identity," *AEM Education and Training,* 2019.

McCullough, L.B., Coverdale, J.H., Chervenak, F.A., "Trustworthiness and professionalism in medicine," *Academic Medicine,* 2020.

Kinsinger, F.S., "The Set and Setting: Professionalism Defined," *Journal of Chiropractic Humanities,* 2005.

Kirk, L.M., "Professionalism in medicine: definitions and considerations for teaching," *Proceedings of Baylor University Medical Center,* 2007.

Al-Rumayyan, A., Van Mook, W.N.K.A., Magzoub, M.E. *et al.,* "Medical professionalism frameworks across non-Western cultures: A narrative overview," *Medical Teacher,* 2017.

Silver, J.K., Cuccurullo, S., Weiss, L.D. *et al.,* "The vital role of professionalism in physical medicine and rehabilitation," *American Journal of Physical Medicine and Rehabilitation,* 2020.

CHAPTER 2

Ethics for Professionals

One does not need be a biomedical ethicist to practise with integrity, but all caregivers must practise ethically.

Ethics and professionalism are integrally linked. All practitioners share the responsibility to have currency with the ethics and virtues of care, because professionals serve the public, and members of the public have great personal needs they give over to their professional. The Social Contract clearly sets out what members of the public expect from the professions.

When consulted, a practitioner uses his or her specialized education, skills and experience to help a patient during a time of need, thereby relieving their distress.

When patients present for care they express great concern, as their needs cause anxiety, discomfort and often hardship. Pain impairs one's ability to carry on with normal activities of daily living and work tasks.

The primary and pre-eminent reason the public demands that caregivers practice with a solid ethical compass is protection. The power differential means, first and foremost, the vulnerable one, the patient, is to be protected from the powerful one, the practitioner.

Your regulator, a representative of your colleagues and peers, ensures protection of the public through standards of practice, guidelines and investigation of alleged misconduct. Of significance, in protecting the patient, the caregiver can enjoy protection from allegations of incompetence or abuse. This appreciation of the professional's ethical responsibilities helps ensure both parties' expectations are met.

Power, Protection and Trust

The Social Contract between the professions and society gives practitioners a status whereby we are held to higher standards. Professionals have significant power. Any misuse or abuse may cause significant harm.

Patient vulnerability may be understood as powerlessness; temporarily giving over one's personal power to the professional. (The informed consent process honors and respects patient autonomy; a convention based on the power differential.) In providing care, because professionals are trustworthy, the concept of "believe in us," *credat emptor*, applies. This is why society gives us extraordinary powers and privileges. This trust rests on our commitment to hold ourselves to higher standards and contrasts with the usual marketplace dictum, *caveat emptor*, buyer beware.

Fiduciary / Fidelity

Use of specialized knowledge and expertise exclusively for the benefit of the patient is known as the "fiduciary covenant."

All professionals share in the obligation to honor this covenant. (Non health care professionals such as lawyers, finance experts and investment agents also have a fiduciary responsibility.) We are duty-bound to put clients' needs above our own. Both fidelity and fiduciary share the word root *fidere*, which means loyalty and trust. Actions matter and deeds speak. We profess to use our expertise to benefit

others, subordinating our own interests and desires; this part of the
Social Contract's "deal."

Professional Standards

Western culture has evolved dramatically over generations. It is now
fashionable to believe that notions of right and wrong are personal,
subjective and relative to the situation at hand.

Known as *moral relativism,* this "I'm free to choose whatever I want'
approach to life allows anyone to designate themselves as morally
acceptable, and above criticism. Judging another's opinions and behaviors is considered intolerant and not congruent with our contemporary culture's way of thinking.

At one time, the concept of conscience guiding one to always do
right was considered useful and valid. This is flawed. Conscience is difficult to quantify. Broadly it may be defined as that faculty to determine when we are guilty of a moral offence. Conscience, formed by
our family of origin and culture, is then directly linked with feelings of
right and wrong, shame and guilt.

Growing up in a time of moral relativism means that standards
of right and wrong vary from one person to the next and cannot be
trusted in the context of professional standards.

Because we are beholden to protect the patient, high standards are
essential. This is the primary reason why all professions have written
codes of conduct and ethics: protection of the public. If the changes
in society's moral standards affected the professions, there would be
an erosion of the high standards demanded of professionalism as set
out under the Social Contract. These standards protect the public by
ensuring the highest level of trustworthiness.

Ethics vs Morals

While these words seem interchangeable, they are separate and distinct. Morals provide a broad basis for our understanding of right and wrong; this emerging from our family of origin, community and culture. Ethics, predicated on an understanding of right and wrong, is applied morality to specific groups, professions and clinical situations. Every profession displays a code of ethics. More recently new disciplines have been codified as legitimate profession groups. When a group aspires to meet a threshold that reaches the status of "profession", their *first* public messaging is a proclamation of their code of ethics and conduct. It's all about public trust.

Ethics: The "Set"

The ethics of care help us to answer the question: "What should I do?"

These "should" questions are a routine part of a practitioner's busy practice. Without a solid foundation of health care ethics to guide us in handling difficult scenarios, on any given day our judgement may fall short. This may affect a patient's outcome.

Of all the ethical principles that apply to health care, four have been identified as foundational, per the scholarship of bioethicists Beauchamp and Childress: autonomy, beneficence, non-maleficence and justice; the "Big 4." They are best appreciated and applied as a professional's duty to the patient.

Beauchamp & Childress

Professors Thomas Beauchamp (Georgetown University) and James Childress (Virginia) published their first text *Principles of*

Biomedical Ethics in 1979. This heralded the emergence and understanding that bioethics was a distinct domain pertaining directly
to health care decision making. Our understanding of the health
care milieu has been deepened via emerging theses in subsequent
editions. Academicians and clinicians rely on their scholarship
in understanding how to approach both routine and challenging
decisions in health care.

1. AUTONOMY

Autonomy provides that patients are free to make decisions that affect
their needs: free from deceit, duress, constraint or coercion; and are
to be an informed participant in making those decisions. Autonomy
provides respect for personal freedom for both the patient and practitioner alike, that ennobles and professionalizes the clinical encounter.

In health care, embedded in the principle of autonomy is the convention of informed consent. Patients have the right to be properly
informed of their condition, including benefits and risks of the procedures that will be used to assess and treat them. Whether we like it
or not, they make the choices. Practitioners have the responsibility to
ensure the patient or patient's representative has the capacity to give
consent, is provided with sufficient details to choose and eschewing
coercion when making a decision.

Our duty: honor and respect patient choice. It's non-negotiable.

2. BENEFICENCE

Beneficence is the principle of doing good; as much good as possible to
benefit another.

This strong proactive concept aims to remove or prevent a person's problem, always striving to promote the "good, better and best."

Beneficence is not served by partially withholding goods or services in order to prolong or extend services for increased financial gain. Our duty: do good and work hard to do as much good as possible.

3. NON-MALEFICENCE

Non-maleficence means one should never inflict harm or cause damage.

In health care, non-maleficence is embodied in the principle of *Primum Non Nocere*, as found in the Hippocratic Oath: "physician - do no harm". Some patients' problems have solutions that may not be worth proposed treatment when the risk-benefit and cost-benefit ratios are considered. Some of the other ethics including autonomy, veracity and beneficence also apply to such decision making.

We have a duty, in all of our interactions with patients, their loved ones and third parties, not to cause harm.

4. JUSTICE

Justice addresses concepts of fairness and entitlement. (Justice is not the same as equality.)

Our duty to be just is applied to all aspects of proposed care which includes parties far removed from the patient. Fairness is difficult to measure objectively but includes the distribution of goods and services, who receives benefits and to what degree. All patients are to be treated on a fair and respectful basis irrespective of ethnicity, social status or any other type of social or personal uniqueness. This dovetails with the professional's fiduciary obligation. Justice embraces cultural sensitivity and the professional's responsibility to ensure care is optimal regardless of who the patient is, where they have originated and what they may look like.

Justice is not served by using one's position of authority to engage a patient on the basis of financial benefit versus the prudent management of the patient's condition.

Our duty to justice goes beyond a duty to act fairly with patients. Our duty to justice extends to the communities in which we live and work.

The Social Contract speaks to a commitment to serve in our communities for the greater good. A heart for social justice sees the provision of care extend to marginalized and underprivileged communities. This is linked with the professional's role as a Moral Agent and further empowers a practitioner to act justly in all matters in all domains.

5. VERACITY

Veracity refers to the comprehensive, accurate and objective communication of information, and binds the practitioner and patient in an association of truth.

This obligation, based on the respect owed to the patient, is closely linked with fidelity (to fulfill an agreement and keep a promise) and prohibits deceit. This ethical tenet guards trust. We can't expect our patients to trust us if we don't tell them the truth.

We have a duty to ensure all aspects of our work and life, both in and out of the office, advocate for truthfulness.

Misrepresentation occurs in many forms in health care. Regulatory boards and colleges discipline practitioners who, even unintentionally, are less than fulsome in conducting their affairs. Clinical notes and records must be accurate and complete. Billings similarly must be honest and accurate. Because professionals have power, we have a duty to ensure that our signature is used prudently so that patient forms, sick notes, billings and online transactions are truthful.

6. CONFIDENTIALITY

Confidentiality further guards the professional's trustworthiness. While patients surrender personal privacy by granting to their professional privileged information, they do not surrender control over how that information is used.

Confidentiality binds the professional never to divulge privileged patient information to another party, unless permission has been granted by the patient. The trust bond becomes severely weakened if a patient fears unauthorized disclosure. Any non-consenting breach damages the practitioner – patient relationship.

Privacy and Confidentiality

Practitioners are duty bound to protect both privacy and confidentiality. Privacy refers to an individual's expectations to have the personal information they divulge to their health care practitioner guarded carefully and not intruded upon.

Confidentiality is the professional's responsibility in managing this private information. Think of confidentiality as affecting communication between the practitioner and other parties removed from the patient. The list includes office staff, other patients, family members, the patient's employer and third party insurers. Patients control how and when their private information is to be communicated to others.

Clinics using paper charts take care to store them securely so that unauthorized access is prevented. Electronic health records pose no less of a concern. Practitioners who are authorized to manage and administrate clinical affairs hold the same professional duty to protect patient information as much as caring for the patient during the therapeutic encounter. Only those in the patient's "circle of care" may legitimately access confidential information. Unauthorized access is considered by regulators as serious misconduct and subject to professional discipline.

Virtues: The "Setting'

The virtues ask "How should I be?" and "What should I be like?"

Long before a critical mass of the Social Contract emerged, Aristotle advocated for desirable character traits in physicians and how these benefit society. A virtue is part of our character that is good, holds value and benefits others. Our character consists of traits which influence our thinking, words and deeds. Our character is nurtured within family and community. We learn how to be virtuous through our socialization with others. In health care this process is known as Professional Identity Formation. Similar to taking instruction in a sport or learning to play a musical instrument, students acquire those essential professional values from those who have gone before.

Professional Identity Formation

The process whereby a young person enters a professional institution, moves through its educational program and graduates as a health care professional, is termed "Professional Identity Formation." Scholars Richard and Sylvia Cruess have quantified this process in their work. Knowledge, skills and attitudes make up three separate components. While learners are preoccupied with passing exams and completing other educational criteria, they undergo an acculturation process with strict adherence to established norms in attitude and conduct. Deviation from these norms, either during schooling or in practice, necessitates remediation and in rare cases expulsion.

Using the "set and setting" analogy, the ethics of care and the virtues fit together by placing the **set**, the ethics of care, in the **setting**, the virtues.

1. ACCOUNTABILITY

Professionals are accountable in multiple ways: to individual patients, colleagues, governing bodies and society at large. An important part of this accountability is accepting one's duty to serve, sometimes with personal inconvenience, and sometimes with risks when working toward a good outcome. Examples include front line pandemic care practitioners and care of the marginalized or hardship patient.

Accountability and the duty to serve others form the concept of volunteerism in the community where a practitioner resides and works. Professionals number significantly in service clubs, community agencies, hospital boards and in other public organizations large and small.

2. EMPATHY

Empathy is a trait that combines an active regard for another's welfare by modelling an awareness and a response of tenderness and compassion for another's misfortune or suffering.

Closely allied with compassion is respect, this being the essence of humanism, another aspect of professionalism. Individuals have immutable rights and therefore are worthy of respect for their individuality. Compassion and respect are virtues which follow from the ethical tenets of autonomy and justice.

Sympathy, Empathy & Compassion

Empathy and compassion are two virtues regarded as essential for anyone involved in patient care. The public has an expectation that providers are caring and humane. What about sympathy? Does a practitioner need to be sympathetic to the plight of a patient?

Sympathy is sharing the feelings of another. Think of sympathy as personally sharing in another's feelings, "I've been there, too." But empathy is the ability to imagine and understand the feelings of another, without the actual experience of having been there.

Sympathy is personal and often used in the context of grief and loss. If a patient has been involved in a motor vehicle collision and suffered injuries, they need their practitioner to offer an understanding response to their situation. If you yourself had been injured in a crash, you would have the ability to sympathize. This difference matters. Learners are encouraged to be empathetic, not sympathetic. Scholars tell us the three components of empathy are learned: an attitude (affect), a competency (cognitive) and a behavior.

Compassion takes the ability to sense and understand another's plight and moves that to a strong desire to help. Patients need an empathetic response as they share their distress and then need an active response to do something about it. Compassion invokes action.

Sympathy is personal: "I've been there. I know exactly what that's like." Empathy is further removed "I can imagine what you're going through" and Compassion is "I understand what you are going through and am ready to help."

3. EXCELLENCE

Excellence entails conscientious effort; an effort to exceed the ordinary expectations of the patient; an effort to embrace life-long learning, and in effort to give back to the profession. This is a significant part of "professing."

There are many opportunities to participate in governance of your profession. This includes serving on regulatory committees, financially supporting professional programs and community charities, and dedicating time mentoring learners and young professionals.

4. FORTITUDE

Fortitude deals with a firm courage and perseverance despite discomfort, misfortune and even suffering when pursuing a professional task.

Health care history is rich with examples of caregivers and researchers who placed themselves in situations of risk when dealing with unknown threats and diseases. We readily think of health care providers who have chosen to serve the sick and less fortunate in war torn countries and destitute regions. We understand this virtue by observing the challenges faced by pandemic weary front-line providers. These dedicated caregivers exemplify fortitude.

Resilience

Resilience is a desired character trait in health care because of the stressful working conditions learners and caregivers are subject to. Resilience is defined as the ability to handle stress with well managed physical and mental health, the ability to cope despite difficult circumstances and the ability to adapt to adversity. Experts tell us we learn resilience through social supports, physical health, and recreational pursuits. A young practitioner benefits from acquiring resilience because personal and professional challenges are ubiquitous and expected.

5. INTEGRITY

Integrity is the consistent regard for the highest standards of both professional and personal behaviour; being "whole," and not given to duplicity, or a dual character that contrasts one's personal behaviors with professional duties. It speaks of consistency in being fair, straightforward, truthful, dependable and faithful to finish the job. Regulators have authority to investigate alleged misconduct that occurs in activities far removed from patient care.

Honesty & Integrity

These terms go together. Honesty means not telling a lie. Veracity is the commitment to being truthful. Truthfulness invokes a larger context in transparency: detailing length, breadth and depth. Integrity goes one important step further. The meaning of integrity is derived from the mathematical term "integer," a whole number. For health care practitioners this means wholeness; being consistent, avoiding duplicity and upholding the fiduciary convention.

Because professionals are held to higher standards, how we spend our time away from the workplace matters. Inappropriate behavior during time spent away from clinic settings has an effect on patients and colleagues. Misconduct of any kind is incongruent with professional values. Integrity is linked with fidelity, favoring the patient's interests above the practitioner.

6. PRUDENCE

Prudence refers to acting thoughtfully and discretely. A prudent professional is in the moment, mindful of the task at hand, taking care to always think about the implications to the patient and those close to the patient.

Prudence embraces **temperance,** the ability to demonstrate discernment and self control, and is linked with the virtue of compassion and the ethical tenets of veracity and confidentiality.

7. FIDELITY

The professional expresses fidelity by favoring the patient's interests over all others, which is another way to define fiduciary.

While the law cannot force one to practise virtuously, it is the virtues that constitute the most powerful manifestation of one's professionalism. Positioning the set of ethical tenets firmly in the setting of virtues honors and empowers the professional–patient encounter.

Scenarios and Searches

a. Are health care practitioners business people or healers? Identify the tensions between these roles and what strategies best manage and reconcile them.

b. Though the Social Contract is between the *professions* and society, individuals have an obligation to understand its terms and ensure they fulfil their part. What part of you upholding your end of the deal do you see as your biggest challenge?

c. Hippocrates composed "The Oath' thousands of years ago. Read it again noting its currency. How many aspects in the Hippocratic Oath relate to health care in this day and age? (Hint: the professional's power is woven throughout.)

d. The professions and society hold professionals to higher standards compared to members of the public. What does this mean? Is it fair?

You be the judge

A busy multi-disciplinary musculoskeletal rehab corporation, wholly owned by a physical therapist, included multiple clinic staff: two chiropractors, three massage therapists, an athletic therapist and a physiatrist.

A third-party insurer inquired about billings sent out by one of the massage therapists. An investigation confirmed these billings were fraudulent due to excessive fees for massages, and for services billed that never had occurred. The regulatory college's investigation led to disciplinary penalties for the massage therapist including a three month license suspension.

Six months later the clinic owner, the physical therapist, was investigated by their regulator for potential involvement in the scheme. That investigation revealed the following:

- There was no evidence that the physical therapist participated in or even knew of the massage therapist's fraudulent billings;
- The massage therapist was immediately fired when the allegations arose;
- The physical therapist fully cooperated with both colleges' investigations.

The PT college alleged the physical therapist was guilty of supervisory neglect. The college stated all documents, including clinical notes and records and invoices originating from any provider in the clinic were under the auspices and responsibility of the owner, the physical therapist.

The clinic owner insisted that the misconduct was entirely the massage therapist's behavior, and termination occurred immediately.

You be the judge: should the physical therapist be disciplined for the fraudulent billings sent out by the massage therapist?

Further References and Resources

Professors Beauchamp and Childress are the founding scholars in our understanding of how bioethical principles affect patient care.

Beauchamp, Tom, Childress, James, *Principles of Biomedical Ethics,* Oxford University Press, 8th ed., 2019

DuBois, J.M., Kraus, E.M., Mikulec, A.A., Cruz-Flores, S., Bakanas, E., "A humble task; restoring virtue in an age of conflicted interests," *Academic Medicine,* 2013.

Coulehan, J., "On Humility," *Annals of Internal Medicine,* 2010.

Cruess, R.L., Cruess, S.R., Boudreau, J.D. *et al.*, "A schematic representation of the professional identity formation and socialization of medical students and residents: a guide for medical educators," *Academic Medicine,* 2015.

Kinsinger, F.S., "Beneficence and the Professional's Moral Imperative," *Journal of Chiropractic Humanities,* 2009.

Stone, E.G., "Evidence-based medicine and bioethics: implications for health care organizations, clinicians, and patients," *The Permanente Journal,* 2018.

CHAPTER 3

Boundaries and Behaviors

Boundaries can be your best friend. Knowing how to set and maintain a healthy patient boundary allows caregiver and patient to enjoy a safe interaction.

The relationship between you, the professional and the other party, your patient, is by definition and practice different from interactions with friends and family. The contrast is so significant, what may seem a minor indiscretion may result in harm to an unsuspecting patient and negative consequences for others, including the practitioner.

Boundaries change from one person to the next, and may differ from one situation to the next. For example, you may feel comfortable with something another person finds intrusive and objectionable. You reveal more of yourself to a friend than you ever would to a patient. You may find a certain joke to be offensive that a friend finds quite humorous.

Inappropriate behavior by a health professional sometimes results in disciplinary proceedings. Misconduct causes unpleasant and even long-lasting *sequelae*. The heart of the problem lies in the potent combination of the position of power held by the professional contrasted with patient vulnerability and weakness.

While the literature suggests some specialties are more prone to boundary violations, few disciplines are exempt from this concern. All caregivers share some risk due to the close physical working quarters and the necessity of touch during physical examination and treatment.

For disciplines that feature close physical contact, it is imperative that learners are aware of this potent crucible of patient vulnerability and the professional's power. Clinical procedures must be carried out with prudent discernment. Empathetic and attentive listening skills combined with the skilful eliciting of relevant information, especially when focusing on an area of complaint, will affect some patients who may themselves be vulnerable and seek more than just expert care.

Boundary Defined

Boundaries protect us by keeping us separate and distinct from each other. Think of a boundary as an unseen layer or invisible coating that all persons have. This is the separation between two people, offering protection from potentially harmful situations. Boundaries regulate our inter-personal interactions and provide personal control, privacy and security. We constantly monitor our boundary to allow some things in and to keep other things out.

There is no such thing as a boundary that is rigid, "set in stone" and never altered. Because we interact differently with different people, and sometimes differently with the same individual depending on the setting, we are continually observing and regulating our boundary awareness. Context is key.

Each person in a relationship, health care or personal, is entitled to set and maintain their own boundaries. While in the professional – client interaction each party is entitled to expect the other to respect established boundaries, it is always the professional who is responsible for managing the interaction.

While boundaries are not visible, it is easy to create a visual image for a patient through our dress. A professional uniform, clinic jacket or business attire all serve this purpose well. Learners wear clinic attire when observing or treating patients.

Practitioners can also take care to meet with patients only in a clinical setting, and not, for example, at social gatherings, a restaurant or a patient's residence. The use of gowns, draping and examination gloves all depict a visual barrier.

The Slippery Slope

The fiduciary covenant mandates that professionals are to always, and without exception, use their expertise for the benefit of the client. Everything we say and do in the presence of the patient is part of the clinical encounter. Much of the practitioner - patient interaction features dialogue between two individuals. The biopsychosocial model of care, taught in all disciplines, humanizes this interaction whereby both individuals' values and expectations are considered in facilitating the goal of a good outcome.

Historically, professional groups have used a Slippery Slope model to warn their members about becoming overly friendly. This approach uses proscriptive terminology: "don't do this" and "watch out for that" and "you're dancing on a slippery slope; so take care not to lose your footing." Because boundary maintenance is nuanced and contextual, there will be times when a discerning practitioner will need to shift to a more rigid slippery slope model, as some patients' interactions cause concern.

Nuance and context do not equate with ambiguity. The practitioner, holding the position of power, is always responsible for a safe and secure encounter. The one absolute proscription every jurisdiction forbids is any romantic and sexual activities with patients. Regulatory

Boards, Colleges and Councils take these allegations seriously, and if proven, mete out severe penalties.

As an alternative to the Slippery Slope model, some scholarship suggests good patient care encourages the professional to intentionally cross a boundary in order to enable a more optimal healing encounter. Stated differently, patient care consists of two individuals (practitioner and patient) in the clinical encounter; with these two experiencing an interpersonal interaction. Because the reagent is the power differential, the repeating message is that the responsibility for prudent management falls to the "power party", the practitioner.

Crossing & Violating

A boundary crossing is defined as words or actions that, strictly quantified, are not part of the therapeutic encounter's clinical domain. We cross with chit-chat. This includes the weather, a favoured sports team's winning or losing record or any other mutually shared interest. Such conversation is safe and benign because little personal information is disclosed to the patient. (Conversely, patients *are* expected to share personal details with their practitioner; this, part of the power imbalance.)

A violation is a boundary crossing that causes harm, or has the potential to cause harm. The most common example is a practitioner disclosing personal information that ought not be conveyed to a patient; usually disclosure of a strained relationship with the practitioner's significant other. Other examples include offering to use the power position to advocate for the patient where such advocacy is considered inappropriate.

Safe (and fun) crossing examples include the occasion when a patient offers a gift, a small token of appreciation. Another might be you offering an affirming hand shake, pat on the back or even a brief hug. There is minimal risk to the patient and such a well-placed caring gesture strengthens the practitioner – patient relationship. This nurtures trustworthiness and practitioners are encouraged to seek opportunities to cross safely.

Conversely, violations erode patient trust.

Boundary violations are crossings that harm the patient (or staff member) or have the potential to cause harm. Examples range from sexualized humor (patient or colleague), a practitioner's indiscrete sharing of personal information, to the most egregious forms of sexual abuse. These offer no benefit to the patient and breech the professional's fiduciary covenant to always favor patient interests. The scholarship is unequivocal that boundary violations never benefit a patient or enhance a therapeutic relationship. Such misconduct serves to satisfy a practitioner's unmet personal needs.

Regulatory boards, colleges and councils use their public record to report member discipline. This serves two important purposes. As under the Social Contract's terms, society is made aware of the open and transparent mechanism of the regulator's primary function to protect the public. Secondly, members of the profession are made aware of the consequences from such violations, and how misconduct causes harm.

Patient Vulnerability

Under the terms of the Social Contract between the professions and society, the practitioner occupies the "power, trust and authority" position. Patients are weak because they are vulnerable, and are vulnerable because they are needy.

Patients present with problems they cannot manage on their own. Symptoms, impaired function, disability, the inability to self-care and anxiety all heighten an urgent need for resolution. Ordinary members of society cannot manage themselves well enough to survive every circumstance in life. As patients we have finite limits on both time and the ability to solve our problems.

We are forced to accept our vulnerability and become dependent on a health care professional, who we give ourselves over to in a time of crisis. This is the essence of vulnerability, in giving up personal control and seeking help. The more urgent our need, the greater our vulnerability.

Being worthy of trust is paramount. We need to place our trust in one who is sensitive to our vulnerability, and acts exclusively in our best interest. Protection of our vulnerability combined with clinical expertise nurtures trustworthiness.

Other Social Contracts

There are other contracts in society for the greater good. All are predicated on a society's shared responsibility to honor and protect a community, a jurisdiction's constitution, order and good governance. Parents have a uniquely powerful position and responsibility. Power is accorded to parents and legal guardians to nurture and protect children. In health care decision-making, since infants and children lack the capacity to consent, it is the parent or guardian who acts as the decision maker.

Educators and those mentoring students hold power over learners and take care not to use their position for personal benefit. Likewise, employers are similarly empowered in their interactions with their employees, subject to employment laws and regulations.

Law enforcement and our justice system afford great power to police, prosecutors and judges. Society advocates for peace, order and protection with this power subject to legislation.

As health care professionals, society gives us great power, and we have an unending obligation to use our power for good by meeting patients' needs, thereby making a positive difference in people's lives. This powerful authority, given to us in trust, serves the communities we live and work in.

The professional's work is sanctioned by governments through laws and regulation. Legislation legitimizes a profession and mandates regulation. Regulation provides many functions in the affairs of a profession. All disciplines share one key maxim: protection of the public. This is *the* primary role of every American state board, Canadian provincial regulatory college and regulatory council in the United Kingdom.

Gender Concerns

In most cultures there is a difference in how we understand subtleties of power. Males often view power as an inherent part of their gender and sexuality. Since our society confuses love, sex and intimacy, dominant, controlling and abusive behaviors may be manifested by the misuse of a practitioner's position.

This is noted when reading reports from regulators. Disciplinary proceedings regarding sexual abuse most commonly reveal male misconduct towards females. However this is not an exclusive pattern as some professions have disciplined female practitioners for sexual abuse, particularly in establishing a romantic relationship without having first observed their regulator's "cooling off" term.

All of the boundaries in the practitioner-patient relationship exist for the patient's safety and protection. Notwithstanding this core intent in protecting the patient, the practitioner also derives enormous benefit from the establishment and maintenance of functional boundaries, as they provide safe limits on what is expected in the encounter.

Altering these limits produces ambiguity, uncertainty and confusion from the patient's perspective.

The take-home message is reassuring: when the patient is protected, the practitioner is protected.

Who's in Charge?

While both parties share the expectation of mutual respect, it is the exclusive responsibility of the practitioner to set and maintain a functional boundary. Violations may be difficult to initially discern, as they are often part of an ongoing process rather than an isolated event. They range on a continuum from minor mistakes to major transgressions.

Every practitioner encounters a flirtatious patient and one that acts out. Most patients have "read the book", know how to behave and make patient care a rewarding and enjoyable pursuit. A small minority cause concern. When confronted with a difficult patient, adopting the Slippery Slope model of interaction should be the first response and then referring such a patient to another practitioner is a recommended course of action.

Touching

Almost all health care disciplines use assessment and treatment involving protocols that touch patient anatomy. The manual care disciplines feature palpation as the primary methodology for assessment and care. Some specialties' scopes focus on intimate anatomy and function. Patients expect to disrobe for many types of care but have the expectation that their professional will take great care to protect their vulnerability with proper use of gowns, draping, examination gloves and chaperone assistants.

Types of Touch

Touching in health care is divided into two categories: intentional and non-intentional. Irrespective of what anatomical area is palpated, the practitioner is duty-bound to employ ongoing communication to ensure the patient is aware of what to expect *and* gives consent. Some professions offer their practitioners a specialized consent protocol when proposed care necessitates touching a sexualized anatomical area.

Statute and case laws identify buttock, genitalia and the female breast as the three sexualized anatomical areas. This means when a practitioner makes direct contact, even legitimately in the clinical setting, *but without patient consent,* the threshold of criminal sexual assault may be reached. Some health care practitioners have been found guilty of sexual assault for touching a sexualized area over top of patient clothing; no disrobing having occurred.

1. Intentional, compassionate and therapeutic touching is beneficent, caring and facilitates healing.
2. Conversely, intentional non-clinical touching is malevolent, harmful and may reach the threshold of criminality.

Non-intentional touch may be accidental or incidental.

3. *Accidental* touch is unplanned and brief. Examples include brushing up against a patient while assisting them move on an examination table or in making some other inadvertent contact. It is brief. With these scenarios it might be appropriate to offer a brief apology "Oops, sorry about that" or something similar.
4. *Incidental* touch may be routine and is commonly on the back of the practitioner's hand or outside edge of the thumb or fingers while the practitioner is palpating or treating. Wise practitioners include this reality when engaging the patient in the consent process. Accidental and incidental touch are not misconduct and do not form the basis for discipline.

Types of Boundary Violations

Boundaries are violated when one party crosses the line by doing or saying something that causes harm or has the potential for harm. Patients react to violations. Physical reactions include tightening in the throat, stomach, upper back and neck and increased cardiac and respiration rates. Some withdraw and become non-responsive. There may be no obvious outward response but anxiety, confusion and anger are common when a practitioner has attempted to sexualize a clinical encounter.

Most cases that end up in disciplinary proceedings begin with excessive self-disclosure on the part of the practitioner. This occurs by talking about personal problems, establishing a dual relationship, giving or receiving gifts and other grooming behaviors. Unchecked this leads to increasing personalization, use of terms of endearment, and discussing a patient's physical features or lifestyle. This inappropriate intimacy is the precursor for overt sexual behaviors.

Seeing patients in social settings, dual relationships and the use of alcohol or drugs during the encounter all constitute high risk boundary behaviors.

Self-Disclosure vs. Personalizing

Knowing how much to say to your patient is a key part of learning the art of practise. It is essential for you to safely connect with your patient. The subtlety in setting and maintaining a functional boundary is knowing how to manage the interaction. Connecting is one skill but then being able to distance yourself from the patient is also an important part of managing boundaries.

Safe self-disclosure is communicating personal information that is benign, non-threatening and may enhance the professional-client relationship. For example, proclaiming yourself a New York Yankees fan, or a lover of classical music, may enhance your ability to relate to a patient. Avoid anything controversial.

Offering supportive words to a new mother nursing a colicky infant, by relating your own personal experiences as a new mom, may serve to strengthen the trust bond you are establishing with that patient. Appropriate self-disclosure is always done prudently so as to remove any uncertainty or confusion.

Personalizing is self-disclosure to a degree that damages the professional encounter and harms both parties. This is a violation and takes the form of the practitioner discussing personal issues with the patient. First, it renders the professional vulnerable by having revealed information of a deeper personal nature that should not be shared. It causes the patient confusion and apprehension. Some patients will withdraw and discharge themselves from care. Others will perceive this as an invitation to engage further thinking their practitioner has now invited them to meet on more than just a clinical playing field.

The dysfunction is the reversal in caregiving. The position of power is given over to the patient, so the patient ends up trying to be a caregiver to the practitioner. Both parties are now at risk and forms the precursor to illegitimate emotional and physical intimacy.

Transition Zone

The Transition Zone refers to the time between finishing a patient's care and the practitioner or patient vacating the treatment area. Wise practitioners manage it well. Practitioners who have been found guilty of misconduct have often violated boundaries during this time. Students are warned to take care with the Transition Zone and learn how to give patients an appropriate "good-bye."

Humor

Most people enjoy a good joke. Some know how to tell one. Practitioners are warned to take great care with humor when engaging with office staff and patients. This is part of boundary maintenance. Knowing that humor is one type of boundary crossing, at what point will a patient (or office colleague), find a joke inappropriate and therefore a violation?

Health corporations, hospitals, employers and regulators receive complaints of offensive and inappropriate humor with work colleagues. A defense of not having an intent to cause offence or harm is not credible.

A safe guideline: if you can take a joke home and share it around the supper table with family present, go for it. Otherwise, tread carefully. If in doubt, don't.

Dual Relationships

Professional groups strongly advise against the treatment of family members. Some jurisdictions forbid it. There is good reason for this, and it is entirely about providing quality care.

A dual relationship occurs when a patient has another type of relationship with their practitioner. Commonly this is a social or business relationship. The list includes friends, acquaintances from church or little league, employees and professional colleagues. If a practitioner enters into a different relationship (commonly social) with an existing patient, a dual connection is established. The elephant in the room is always the power differential.

Regulators will investigate practitioners for non-emergency treatment of family members, with allegations usually originating from other providers. This episodic care is considered sub-optimal as clinical notes and records are rarely kept. Wise caregivers recognize the inherent danger is in compromising the therapeutic encounter and providing a marginalized standard of care. Family members deserve better.

The best care is rendered when there are no strings or influences affecting either party. While sometimes tolerated, dual relationships are to be avoided.

False Intimacy

Health care practitioners are more at risk of violating a patient's boundaries when they themselves are unbalanced in their personal life. The "HALT" quartet of Hungry, Angry, Lonely and Tired is used as a teaching strategy in many rehab settings. It refers to being self-aware and maintaining a healthy mind, body and spirit. When we are not at our best, we are more vulnerable to our personal idiosyncratic dysfunctions and potential self- destructive behaviors. We see this with patients all the time. Why would we think we're immune?

Since by human nature we are wired for intimacy, designed to connect with others, it is essential that we satisfy our deepest and most intimate personal needs outside of and quite apart from our professional work. When a practitioner experiences difficulty in relationships with those who are closest, particularly relationship problems with their significant other, the practitioner's vulnerability looms large, as intimacy needs will be met, and patients are at risk.

The most dangerous situation is when both practitioner and patient have significant unmet personal needs. Knowing that the professional acts as a caretaker, boundary violations pervert the role of caretaker by having the professional adopt the vulnerable position. A practitioner at risk, out of balance, with unmet personal needs, is especially vulnerable with a patient who, for whatever dysfunctional reason, may want to assert him or herself in the caretaking role.

Transference

Patients frequently develop what is termed role transference toward their practitioner. Subconsciously the patient transfers to the professional feelings and behaviors from previous personal relationships. Transference may take the form of the patient interacting with and seeing the professional as a pseudo-parent, adopting aberrant or child like behaviors. Like a child these behaviors may be acted out as compliant or adversarial. Examples include flirting, offering gifts, unquestioning acceptance, behaving seductively or refusing to pay an account.

This is a difficult concept for young learners to comprehend while still training. Experienced practitioners see it routinely. While practitioners in the psychotherapeutic disciplines seek to use transference as part of therapy, all practitioners have to manage transference as part of boundary setting and maintenance. Wise practitioners know when to move the patient to a rigid Slippery Slope interaction.

Countertransference

Countertransference is the practitioner transferring his or her feelings to the patient in response to the patient's transference. A practitioner may be quite unaware of this and be vulnerable to the transference behaviors of the patient. This translates into each party being co-dependent on the other.

Countertransference can manifest itself in different ways. Examples include entering into a dual relationship with a client (such as a business venture); assuming an arrogant or condescending posture in order to accentuate the professional's position of power; or acting on a romantic desire with a patient.

"But My Patient Consented"

It is not possible for a patient to be a willing and consenting partner in any type of romantic or sexual relationship with their caregiver. This is entirely because of the power differential and the unlevel playing field. A patient is not in a position to give consent. Appellate case law has upheld this prohibition in many jurisdictions when a practitioner argued that his patient was a consenting adult with decisional capacity.

Despite this being forbidden in all professions, it happens. A sexual relationship is disgraceful, dishonorable and unprofessional. It brings dishonor to one's profession and is the severest kind of ethical violation. Abused patients frequently need counselling assistance to recover from such abuse. License suspension and revocation routinely follow.

Harassment vs. Abuse vs. Assault

While some use these words interchangeably, there are differences. Your Board, College or Council carefully articulates what category specific behaviors fall into. All three constitute professional misconduct.

Sexual Harassment refers to unwelcomed talk of a sexual nature, usually by someone in an authority position. Workplace settings are associated with sexual harassment. It is not uncommon for regulators to discipline practitioners who have mistreated employees or co-workers. Gratuitous terms of endearment and unwanted workplace touching is harassment.

Sexual Abuse refers to verbal or physical behavior of a sexual nature by a regulated professional. Jurisdictions provide explicit details on what constitutes sexual abuse. Because regulation is predicated on legislation, jurisdictions may differ on both definitions and penalties for the types and severity of sexual abuse.

Sexual Assault refers to behaviour that reaches a criminal threshold. Under law, intentional, non-consensual and non-clinical touching of sexualized anatomical areas constitutes sexual assault. No patient ever consents to be abused or assaulted. While a criminal charge is rare, regulators monitor court proceedings when a member is on trial for sexual assault. Even when acquitted on the criminal charge, practitioners are commonly found to have reached the lower threshold of sexual abuse and subject to discipline.

A Word on Dating Patients

Don't.

It is improper, irregular and highly unethical to invite a patient out on a date. When new to practice, a patient may ask you out. Expect it. Patients don't realize they are asking you to breach your profession's code of ethics, but you do.

While most jurisdictions allow for a patient to be formally discharged from care to permit a potential romantic relationship, you must always act in your patient's best interests. Refer your patient formally to a colleague, and then comply with the required wait time before acting on your romantic desires. Regulators discipline members who are non-compliant in waiting out the required term.

Recovering Lost Boundaries

Practitioners sometimes realize they may have participated in a more minor type of boundary violation. It is entirely possible to recover from minor boundary violations by crossing back. Minor indiscretions can usually be dealt with by the practitioner acknowledging the change in dynamics and inappropriate dialogue, and then asserting future encounters will be professionally focussed.

Gross misconduct is difficult to resolve. This requires assistance from a third party, and not always with a happy outcome for the principal participants. Disciplinary penalties include suspension of one's license to practice, remediation for the professional and recovery of costs from the investigation plus costs for patient counseling.

Revocation, losing one's license to practice, constitutes the final last word on a profoundly sad situation.

Scenarios and Searches

a. Boundary maintenance is contextual and always nuanced. Brainstorm what self-disclosure might look like between different patients. For example, how might your *crossing* contrast between a 25 year old patient compared with a 65 year old? Discuss other types of scenarios. What are the obvious concerns? What subtleties can you identify? Another example is the patient with body art, tattoos. Should a practitioner engage in talk about a patient's tattoo? What types of comments would fall into both the crossing and violating categories?

b. Locate both your regulator and professional association publications searching for those behaviors that constitute sexual abuse. If your jurisdiction has yet to publish these, source them from a different profession or jurisdiction.

c. Boundary violations may be initiated by the patient. If a patient becomes overly interested in the practitioner's personal life with intrusive questions and inappropriate comments, how should this be dealt with? Should patients routinely be provided your personal contact number?

d. Health care practitioners are reminded to take care when treating the "attractive" patient. Absent is anything at the other end of the continuum, the "repulsive" patient. Discuss this rare situation beginning with what types of distinguishing characteristics such a patient might present with. Make it personal identifying what differences in others you like and dislike, and what might impress you as repulsive. Based on the ethics and virtues of care, how is such a patient is to be dealt with?

You be the judge

A psychotherapist in a drug and alcohol rehab facility was under investigation regarding a lady who had been an inpatient for 8 weeks. He was one practitioner in her circle of care and had spent extra time chatting with her when he was off duty. He gave her his private number so she could keep in touch. Both were single.

Five days after discharge she contacted him. She had been searching for a small apartment to rent and was almost out of money. He offered her the basement in his residence at no cost. Both agreed it would be temporary. Soon they began to share meals and movies. Within a week they engaged in flirtatious behavior which soon progressed to sexual activity. Two months later they became engaged, and six months later they married. Another psychotherapist at the hospital reported the relationship to the licensing body.

After gathering statements from all of the principals involved, the regulator alleged the psychotherapist had engaged in a series of boundary violations beginning with being too casual and friendly when the patient was still under institutional care, and that it was inappropriate to have contact with her so soon after discharge.

The psychotherapist argued that no inappropriate activity occurred at the hospital, the client was no longer under his care, they both were consenting adults who subsequently married, and now were expecting their first child.

You be the judge: Did the friendly talks while the patient was hospitalized constitute a boundary crossing? Boundary violation? After discharge, what was the status of the former patient? What about inviting her to move into the basement? Was there anything about the establishment of the sexual relationship that is contrary to professional standards of practice?

Further References and Resources

In whatever jurisdiction you intend to practice in, both the licensing body and professional association have already published guidelines on setting boundaries.

Before delving into the scholarly literature, read their guidelines and recommendations first. Compare "yours" with a few other professions. On establishing romantic relationships, note the referral requirements and strict time-lines. Many of the psychotherapeutic disciplines proscribe a lifetime prohibition in romancing a former patient.

Arroll, B., Allen, E.C.F., "To self-disclose or not self-disclose? A systematic review of clinical self-disclosure in primary care," *British Journal of General Practice,* 2015.

Kinsinger, F.S., Sutton, W., "Chiropractic Leadership in the Eradication of Sexual Abuse," *Journal of the Canadian Chiropractic Association,* 2012.

Manfrin-Ledet, L., Porche, D.J., Eymard, A.S., "Professional boundary violations: a literature review," *Home Healthcare Now,* 2015.

Morse, D.S., McDaniel, S.H., Candib, L.M., *et al., "'Enough about me, let's get back to you': physician self-disclosure during primary care encounters," Annals of Internal Medicine,* 2008.

Nieva, H.R., Ruan, E., Schiff, G.D., "Professional-patient boundaries: a national survey of primary care physicians' attitudes and practices," *Journal of General Internal Medicine,* 2020.

Sawyer, S., Prescott, D., "Boundaries and dual relationships," *Sexual Abuse: a Journal of Research and Treatment,* 2011.

Sossauer, L., Schindler, M., Hurst, S., "Vulnerability identified in clinical practice: a qualitative analysis," *BMC Medical Ethics,* 2019.

CHAPTER 4

Conflicts of Interest & Integrity

There may not be a more desired virtue for a practitioner to model and uphold, than integrity.

Having integrity means that one takes care to make wise choices, with words and actions that nurture and strengthen the patient's trust-bond, always actively pursuing the best for the patient. This recurring theme was first articulated as a principle in Chapter 1. The centrality of it never fades.

A person of integrity has the reputation they can be trusted. Since actions speak louder than words, how we act is more important than what we say, and must equate to our words. Both the concept and significance of integrity are richly woven into everything that occupies our work, with integrity forming the most significant part of the *setting* of professionalism in Chapter 2.

Integrity

Integrity means to be whole, complete and consistent in word and deed. It means being ever truthful with colleagues, patients and others, and honors high standards of behavior both in private life and in public. This wholeness of person gives an inner sense of serenity in knowing that we are living well and doing right. And when the professional falls short, for whatever reason, as everyone does on occasion, the response is a genuine expression of contrition, humility and when appropriate, making amends.

Integrity is a word that is often used in the public domain. Members of the public respond favorably to this character trait when demonstrated in others. We desire to have other people that we know and interact with, be people of integrity. Politicians and others in the public eye particularly like to use this word, but any objective scrutiny of behaviors would reveal that many in the public spotlight do not act with integrity.

Professionalism demands that what we say is wholly true, and that what we do completely agrees what we say. This nurtures and maintains trustworthiness.

Starting in middle school math classes, we learned an integer was a whole number. It shares the same word root as integrity. Duplicity refers to a dual character; acting professionally at work but not necessarily when enjoying leisure time pursuits.

Duplicity is hypocrisy. Saying one thing and then doing another demonstrates untrustworthiness. Such individuals cannot be trusted. We readily see examples, as our current culture's moral relativism is antithetical to concepts of absolutes.

Parents guide their children in gaining an understanding of what a reputation is, and how this affects a child's interactions with friends, neighbors and teachers. We all desire a good reputation. A reputation is slow to build and nurtured over time. In the era of social media, one's reputation is at risk with even one momentary indiscretion.

Our reputation is based entirely on how we conduct ourselves: our speech, our actions and reactions. Our reputation then becomes an integral part of defining our character. A reputation can be unalterably changed in a momentary lapse, through one unfortunate occurrence. We witness these occurrences in social media and news reports.

While we all enjoy personal liberties in making choices in the things we say and do, the resulting consequences of our actions are rarely under our control. Consequently, our integrity should affect our personal choices, keeping in mind the rewards of a good reputation.

When parents trust an adolescent, privileges are much more likely than when there is a problem with distrust. For the professional, a good name and an honorable reputation are more valuable than any other asset. Under the auspices of the Social Contract and from the public's perspective, integrity is automatically accorded to professionals (it comes with the territory), but like a valuable commodity, is to be protected.

In other words, we start out with a good reputation, and are obligated to maintain the honor of the high calling of the profession and the high standards of professionalism. It is because of this that inappropriate conduct from even just one careless practitioner can cause harm to the reputation of the whole profession. This may not seem fair, but is reality.

Integrity is expressed in these three virtues.

1. COMMITMENT

Commitment means to keep your word by being reliable. It conveys more than just words, but denotes actions. We trust the people we enter into a contract with to fulfil the terms. Like us, they think through the situation, weigh and balance all options, and then commit themselves accordingly. There is a shared responsibility to weigh the risks and benefits before signing the deal. We honor our commitments by keeping our word.

2. FORTHRIGHTNESS

Forthrightness means that what we say and how we say it conveys our intent clearly without being dodgy or deceptive. Communication in a highly politicized culture bathed in social media, poses challenges. Since tolerance and forthrightness are not mutually exclusive, health practitioners need to maintain the reputation of being honest and true in thought, word and deed.

3. STEADFASTNESS

Steadfastness means to work hard and uninterrupted in the face of obstacles, distractions and criticism. The professional's steadfastness is seen in upholding excellence, fortitude and discernment, and no part of laziness, fickleness or fanaticism.

How does steadfastness fit with integrity? By continuously acting on three things: discerning right from wrong; demonstrating use of this knowledge in a caring way, and following up with action steps.

Conflicts of Interest

A conflict of interest occurs when the primary interest, the patient, is interfered with by another interest; one favoring the professional, directly or indirectly. This secondary interest influences the objectivity with which the practitioner provides care for the patient, thereby threatening the fiduciary relationship.

All of us have routine conflicts of interest in our work that are legitimately considered minor and rarely lead to negative consequences.

For example, practitioners rarely care for patients after regular office hours. This is an example of a conflict that may not be in a patient's immediate best interests. It competes with the practitioner's interest in fulfilling family responsibilities. With established time boundaries, after hours emergency appointments tend to disrupt valuable personal time spent with family. Patients get that.

Another example is limiting the amount of time spent with a patient during office visits. Patients understand there are other people waiting for care who must not be unduly delayed. This rarely puts a burden on a patient, and practitioners have no duty to disclose these common conflicts.

Other conflicts of interest are neither minor nor benign.

Conflicts are predicated on the professionals' position of power and trust. The party in the position of power, the professional, has the continuing obligation to exercise professional judgement exclusively for the benefit of the patient, but has a competing secondary interest that benefit the professional providing the service.

These secondary interests all have a detrimental impact on the practitioner-patient relationship and weaken the practitioner's fidelity and the patient's trust.

1. FINANCIAL GAIN

Financial conflicts of interest come in every shape and size, and are recognized as the most common source of conflict in health care. Fee for service billing provides an incentive for many practitioners to use additional diagnostic and therapeutic procedures, even when they don't serve the patient's interests in risk-benefit and cost-benefit considerations.

Health corporations reward an individual practitioner's frugal choices by offering financial bonuses, creating an incentive to limit more expensive procedures. This may not be in the patient's best interests. A patient may be denied a recommended service or procedure based on the desire to save expenses.

Note that many unethical decisions are not deliberative, but occur as unconscious self-serving biases, beyond the realm of intentional choices and often subsumed into an organization's business model.

2. PERSONAL GRATIFICATION

A practitioner with conflict in his or her personal relationships, and who does not take care to guard patient boundaries is at risk for personalizing the relationship. This may lead to engaging in inappropriate behaviors that abuse the client. While not necessarily sexualized, this desire for intimacy creates a conflict by reversing the roles and damages the professional's trustworthiness.

3. PROFESSIONAL FAME

A practitioner's desire to achieve notoriety may manifest itself in behaviors which seek to serve the goals of the practitioner. Conflicts of interest in research are evidenced by those who would conspire to either misappropriate data, misrepresent scholarly activity or withhold recognition where due.

4. PERSONAL PRESTIGE

Practitioners who would prefer to care for a higher socio-economic group and upper-class clientele have a conflicted interest towards a less desirable patient that attends for care. This category of conflict includes business venture dual relationships, which compromises not just that patient's care, but may compromise the care given to other patients as well.

5. LEISURE ACTIVITES

Many a birthing mother with a slow labor has been referred for a Caesarian section due to the impending deadline of the attending physician's tee-off time or some other personal activity.

6. PEER PRESSURE

A professional more concerned about reputation with other colleagues may experience a direct conflict with the needs of the patient. This incentive puts the patient in a subservient position. Refusing a patient adequate diagnostic testing so as to appear discerning and frugal may compromise a patient's health status.

Reluctance to refer to a practitioner outside of the usual comfort zone or scope's usual referral pattern may not be in the patient's best interests. This is more common in some disciplines and includes referral to those practicing the CAM disciplines.

7. EDUCATIONAL COMPETENCIES

Professionals, active in teaching clinics, are at risk for mandating procedures or prescribing other goods and services that serve their student's educational experience, and not necessarily best for the patient.

8. ALLOCATION OF RESOURCES

When resources are scarce or there is an incentive to restrict goods or services, this conflict rears its head in denying or restricting care. Most clinical triage and case management is dependent on resources available. A conflict becomes real when the patient suffers material risk or their condition worsens, as a result of lack of care, which may have been initially compromised by the withholding of optimal goods and services.

Resolving Conflicts

Regulated practitioners have a professional responsibility to disclose. Jurisdictions articulate what situations and scenarios fall under this duty. (See Chapter 5 for further discussion of this professional responsibility.) Since conflicts of interest come in different forms, there is no one, cure-all, action step.

Firstly, the practitioner needs to be aware of the potential for a conflict, and then be able to identify the competing interests. Secondly, the parties are to be notified. The list may or may not include the patient but usually involves other professional colleagues and third party payors.

When disclosure flags a potential conflict, resolutions differ depending on the circumstances. If all parties agree that the conflict is manageable and that untoward influence may be mitigated, the practitioner is given the green light. Should one party be unwilling to proceed, the patient (or client in some non-practitioner-patient cases) is either referred elsewhere or handled differently.

Practitioners are cautioned to take care when entering into any type of dual relationship with patients and are to avoid treatment and especially billings for immediate family members. Treating family members gives rise to many types of conflicts and regulators concern themselves with allegations of this loss of objectivity. While there may not have been harm done, the primary role of all regulators is protection of the public.

Misrepresentation

Misrepresentation comes in many forms in health care. The published literature reports benevolent deception; honoring a palliative patient's request to withhold details of a poor prognosis. A practitioner has no such duty to adhere to facts in this rare situation.

Practitioners profess communicating truthfully. There are five ways in which adherence to the truth may be compromised.

1. All communication with patients, colleagues and staff is to fully adhere to the facts. Anything less than fulsome thoroughness has a negative effect on workplace colleagues which may then compromise patient safety. Hospitals and other employers have an expectation that staff and workers honor this virtue.

2. Regulatory boards, colleges and councils demand their members take great care in completing annual re-licensure. Practitioners are to disclose any potential barriers to delivery of care that may affect their fitness to practice, including physical and mental health concerns, police involvement and criminal charges. Professional licensure in other disciplines and jurisdictions must also be disclosed.

3. Fraudulent billings, misuse of the practitioner's signature and pre-signing pads and invoices all constitute misrepresentation.

4. Clinical notes and records are to be accurate. False, incomplete and missing clinical notes and records constitute misrepresentation, as negative consequences tend to be far reaching.

5. For members facing an allegation, any interference or obstruction of the investigation process constitutes misrepresentation.

Besides violating the virtues of honesty and integrity, lying harms multiple parties and breaches the principles of professionalism.

Advocacy vs Objectivity

A practitioner's fiduciary responsibility favors the patient; always an advocate. This commitment to a patient's well being strengthens the trust bond. Part of this convention is the recognition that a practitioner may not be, and should not be, entirely objective towards patients. While this beneficent advocacy is considered a minor conflict of interest, it is accepted as part of good care.

Some patients' problems have a legal component to them. Legal disputes are often dealt with via independent assessments conducted by experts, on referral from a third party. In personal injury cases and other matters of dispute, third party payors and the courts rely on objective and impartial information gathered from expert practitioners. Opinions provided by independent experts form a key part of the medico-legal domain.

Health care practitioners that participate in independent assessments do not establish a caregiving relationship and thus have little fiduciary responsibility toward the person they assess and report on. Their client is whoever pays them to prepare a report, typically an insurance company or lawyer. Those that participate in providing expert opinions are expected to acknowledge their primary interest is not toward the person being assessed. Insurance companies expect their hired assessors to favor the company's corporate interests. Caregivers favor their patient. A case in dispute may end up in a court of law where clinical notes and records along with assessors' reports are made public. Adherence to veracity and conflicts of interest are exposed. Willful blindness and spinning of fact is laid bare under cross examination.

Scenarios and Searches

a. What Conflicts of Interest are most common in your profession?

b. Does your regulatory Board, College or Council publish statutes or guidelines on Conflict of Interest? If you were asked to come up with such a guideline, what would it look like?

c. We have the expectation that patients will trust their caregiver. Explore how one becomes worthy of trust, how this applies in the health care encounter and what limits, if any, protect practitioners and patients?

d. Caring practitioners honor patient requests for sick notes and other kinds of helps. While most are routine others skirt the limits of legitimacy. Consider the following.

A well known patient presents with legal papers seeking permission to access handicapped parking and requests your signature. The details specify, in order to qualify for such a designation, a person must fail to reach a measurable threshold on three separate functional tests. On testing, the patient is functionally sound and fails to meet the threshold on even one of the three.

Explore the issues that arise. How many parties might potentially be involved? Weigh and measure the risks to each party when making your choice. Either you sign the papers despite the patient's failure to qualify, or refuse with an explanation to the patient.

You be the judge

A specialist began a consensual and anonymous online relationship with an individual who lived more than 400 miles away. At first, they chatted. As their relationship progressed, they began to engage in sharing pictures and then engaged in sexual activities, once every week or two. While they both knew what city the other resided in, no personal information, including work status was divulged. At no time did they meet in person.

Two months later the practitioner made a casual comment regarding how a certain health condition is best treated. That led to a disclosure of both the practitioner's specialty and clinic locale. The online relationship ended soon after. Three months later the specialist received a notice from the licensing body. The investigation focused on the establishment of a concurrent clinical and sexual relationship with a patient, and, conduct deemed unbecoming to a health care professional.

The practitioner defended the activity as being entirely unrelated to patient care as the other party was not a patient. The specialist's lawyer argued that the licensing body had no jurisdiction over a member's leisure-time recreational activities.

You be the judge. Was the other party a patient? Does sexting and other online sexual behavior constitute a significant risk to patient safety and the reputation of the profession? Does the regulatory body have control over a member's off-hours activities?

Further References and Resources

"Integrity" is a word commonly used. Re-read its definition to ensure understanding of how and why professionals are held to higher standards. Your licensing body and professional association have already published guidelines on many aspects of practice including proper use of social media, clinical notes and records and conflicts of interest.

Coverdale, J.H., Roberts, L.W., Balon, R. *et al.*, "Professional integrity and the role of medical students in professional self-regulation," *Academic Psychiatry,* 2016.

Decamp, M., "Physicians, social media, and conflict of interest," *Journal of General Internal Medicine,* 2013.

Fink, N.E., "Conflicts of interest and an approach to managing them," *Electronic Journal of the International Federation of Clinical Chemistry,* 2020.

Luft, L.A.M., "The essential role of physician as advocate: how and why we pass it on," *Canadian Medical Education Journal,* 2017.

Tyreman, S., "Integrity: is it still relevant to modern healthcare?" *Nursing Philosophy,* 2011.

CHAPTER 5

Professional Responsibilities

It takes time for a learner to fully appreciate the privilege of providing care and even longer to fully grasp the duties and responsibilities incumbent on professionals. Practitioners are responsible for the custody and care of their patients; but there is more. Responsibility manifests itself beyond the use of clinical skills. Responsibility affects everyone in the professional's circle of influence. As under the Social Contract, our professing positions us as agents of change; change for the better.

Students acquire competencies: attentive listening, focused examination protocols, differentials, and proposing a plan of management. While this all constitutes good care, leadership qualities and responsibilities extend beyond one's clinical acumen.

Leadership and responsibility go hand-in-hand. Being a responsible person draws from the ethics and virtues set out in Chapter 2. Health care professionals have an obligation to act responsibly in all domains, and not just when providing care. This constitutes much of the professions' Social Contract with society, in leading by example.

Do not be dissuaded by what is meant as an obligation to lead. Some may be concerned they may not have what it takes, as they never volunteered for the debating team, student council or community charitable events.

A professional's leadership does not necessitate any of these. Rather it speaks to the heart of the individual in desiring to maintain the highest calling of the fiduciary relationship with the patient. Professionals have a responsibility to make decisions and manage outcomes, optimal or otherwise.

Recall that prudence refers to acting thoughtfully and discretely. A prudent professional is in the moment, mindful of the task at hand, and takes care to consider the implications to the patient and those close to the patient.

Prudence embraces **temperance,** the ability to demonstrate discernment and self control, and is linked with the virtue of compassion and the ethical tenets of veracity and confidentiality.

Responsibility

Most choices in our daily lives have little ethical baggage. What shoes to wear or choice of a food delivery service are routine. Put patients, families of patients and office staff in the mix, and our choices come with consequences.

We are duty-bound to consider how our decision-making affects those around us. Acting responsibly toward others affects everything from our continuing education choices to how we drive and even how late we stay out. We have a duty to act responsibly.

One scholar (Niebuhr) proposes that responsible people exhibit three qualities. These qualities are found under the banner of what all health care practitioners profess:

1. Professionals are able to initiate action,
2. Professionals are able to make an appropriate response to the situation at hand,
3. Professionals are able to account for their actions.

1. INITIATING ACTION

Responsible people take action. They are able to make decisions, well knowing their decisions affect others. As practitioners, we have an inherent responsibility to choose wisely in being discerning, thoughtful and considerate; all predicated on our ability to uphold the virtues of prudence, temperance and integrity. Professionals take care to consider abilities, intellect and emotions. Since health care practitioners are moral agents with power and authority, we have an obligation to take action when needed.

Moral agents are advocates for justice. We profess use of our power position to help the weak and underserved in order to better our society and the communities we live and work in.

2. DISCERNMENT AND RESPONSE

Responsible people react effectively. Knowing how to respond is both reactive and proactive. This seeming contradiction is the ability to take affirmative action in response to a problem; ergo professional work.

Your patient presents with a problem, and you, the practitioner act. The response is proactive; a response to the clinical dilemma. Contrast this with uncivil knee-jerk reactions, which are swift and inflammatory. The essence of the professional's response is discernment.

Discernment

Discernment is the ability to probe deeply and understand what has happened before and may likely happen in the future. We demonstrate discernment when we can be depended on to demonstrate insight, and to know what options are available. Discerning people observe subtleties, nuances and missed clues regarding people, places and things. Demonstrating patience, tolerance and consideration of others facilitates insight and discernment and is another aspect of Moral Agency.

3. ACCOUNTABILITY

Responsible people are accountable for their behavior. Accountability is another virtue that nurtures the professional's relationship to patients and colleagues. Responsible accountability entails more than simply owning up to a decision made. It is predicated on the obligation and responsibility to explain the rationale and background that led to the decision through the decision-making process, and *sequelae*. Accepting accountability and not shifting blame, is a part of civility. Civility is further explored in Chapter 6.

Maturity

The three parts that constitute responsibility equate to what is understood as maturity. Though difficult to quantify, maturity is a commodity that eases learner and practitioner alike, through the rigors of dealing with a complex, hurried, and often uncaring world.

No randomized clinical controlled trial has been published on what makes a person mature. The following seven attributes originated with the late syndicated newspaper columnist Ann Landers. They are as follows:

1. Maturity is the ability to control anger and settle differences without violence and destruction.
2. Maturity is patience. It is the willingness to pass up immediate pleasure in favour of long-term gain.
3. Maturity is perseverance, the ability to sweat out a project

or situation is spite of heavy opposition and discouraging setbacks.

4. Maturity is the capacity to face unpleasantness and frustration, discomfort and defeat without complaint or collapse.

5. Maturity is humility. It is big enough to say "I was wrong." And, when right, not saying "I told you so."

6. Maturity is the ability to make a decision and follow through. The immature spend their lives exploring endless possibilities, and then do nothing.

7. Maturity means dependability, keeping one's word and coming through in a crisis. The immature are masters of the alibi.

Ethical Dilemma

An ethical dilemma is a situation in which there is no obvious automatic, right choice, as two or more ethical principles apply; principles appearing to be in direct conflict. Examples include patient confidentiality competing with a practitioner's legal duty to report to Public Health. Others include a patient requesting goods or services they are not be entitled to. There are many scenarios. While most arise from the clinical domain, it is not the clinical challenge that presents the dilemma, but an overriding ethical principle to best answer the question "What should I do?" These challenge caregivers.

Resolving An Ethical Dilemma

We have a responsibility to make challenging decisions. Some are forced upon us and must be made in an instant, while others simmer over time and require sober reflection. It is the difficult choices that affect our patients, and affect us too.

At some point during professional identity formation learners come to realize that work as a professional is not easy. Some tasks demand our whole being and are stressful.

Being called to professional work differs from other types of employment and is not to be entered into lightly; it's not for everyone.

Not everyone can work within the fiduciary covenant, in nurturing another's trust while maintaining personal integrity and fidelity. Not everyone can be counted on to work in an environment where decisions are made for the benefit of the patient, to the exclusion of the provider. Not everyone can manage multiple responsibilities, with the challenges and difficulties that are incumbent with this calling. Not everyone can become immersed in the most intimate details of a patient's distress while setting a healthy boundary. Without a strong ethical compass and great resilience, these demands are overwhelming.

The scholarly literature provides step-by-step approaches to identify and resolve ethical dilemmas. All share a systematized analysis by identifying the ethical incongruities, considering the parties involved, and how context and other subtleties may affect deliberations. To attempt a logical resolution, it is most important to foresee how each choice causes more or fewer benefits to each party.

This allows the practitioner using the rubric to be one of the players that is factored into the equation. Because ethical dilemmas offer no obvious best choice, two people using the rubric might come up with differing solutions, or may arrive at the same conclusion by using different rationales.

For the learner, to better understand difficult ethical scenarios, spend time with a faculty mentor or experienced practitioner. Clinical experience provides insight into difficult situations that commonly arise in each specialty. Start with a working knowledge of the ethics of care by reviewing the "Big 4" from Chapter 2 and then tease out which ethics are in conflict. Sometimes the best choice is electing to do nothing or, referring the decision-making process to another.

In your clinic setting it may be that a work colleague will be tasked with taking action and you end up being one of the parties affected by the choice. Others land squarely on you, so your reputation as being wholly trustworthy extends to making the best possible decision in difficult circumstances.

3–Step Ethical Dilemma Resolution

1. **Determine the underlying question and ethical incongruity**
   - What are the presenting and underlying questions, problems or issues?
   - Are you responsible for making the decision, or can it be delegated?
   - Who are the main players?
   - What is their relationship to the problem? What are their values and interests? Who are the secondary and tertiary parties?
   - *What primary ethics are in conflict?*
2. **Brainstorm, reflect, weigh and balance the options**
   - Examine the options from the perspective of all players. Most cases include doing nothing, doing a little or doing much more.
   - Weigh and balance each option from the perspective of all of the main players, including the provider.
   - What is the probable impact of each possible course of action? *Who will benefit and whose interests may be overridden by each possible outcome?*
   - What is the probable impact on the institution, the profession and society at large?

- Think the problem through considering the ethical principles behind the options.
- What happened when a similar problem was dealt with before?

3. **Make the decision, Implement and Evaluate**
   - Choose the best course of action that reflects your judgement after considering all of the facts, players and options.
   - *Is this in keeping with the principles of professionalism?*
   - Consider the arguments to counter opposition to your decision, remembering that someone's interests will not be favored.
   - Take the steps necessary to implement the best course of action.
   - Reflect. What would you do differently the next time this dilemma occurs?

Demonstrating Leadership

There are three aspects of leadership that practitioners must be competent in.

- Leadership to the patient and patient's family;
- Leadership to colleagues and the profession as a whole;
- Leadership to the community in which the practitioner lives and works.

An excellent leadership model that health practitioners readily adopt is Robert Greenleaf's Servant Leadership. While this leadership model originated in the business world, it is relevant to health care.

Greenleaf wrote "The servant-leader is servant first. It begins with the natural feeling that one wants to serve. Then conscious choice brings one to aspire to lead. The best test is: do those served grow as persons; do they, while being served, become healthier, wiser, freer, more autonomous and more likely themselves to become servants?"

There are ten characteristics of the servant-leader:

1. LISTENING

No less important than communication, discernment and technical skills that the practitioner requires, this is the deep commitment to listening intently to others.

2. EMPATHY

The servant leader strives to understand and empathize with others. Patients, staff and colleagues need to be accepted and affirmed for their own special and unique spirit.

3. HEALING

While this is obvious for the health care professional, this concept applies to our relationship with the other people we deal with who are not patients. Since we all suffer some brokenness of spirit, servant-leaders recognize that they have an opportunity to help make whole all those they come in contact with.

4. AWARENESS

Starting with self-awareness, this characteristic helps in understanding issues of values, morals and ethics.

5. PERSUASION

This removes one's position of authority, "Because I say so" as the basis for leadership and shifts it to that of persuasion through cooperation, negotiation and consensus building.

6. CONCEPTUALIZATION

The ability to look at a problem, such as that with a patient, a colleague or an organization, not from a day-by-day basis, but from a big-picture view, is the ability to conceptualize.

7. FORESIGHT

Foresight is the characteristic that enables the servant-leader to understand lessons from the past, see the reality of the present and project the likely consequences of the future.

8. STEWARDSHIP

This old-fashioned term means to hold something of value in trust for another. As professionals, we hold our knowledge, skills and experience as a precious commodity in trust for others: the patients we serve, our colleagues with whom we interact and the communities we work in.

9. COMMITMENT TO THE GROWTH OF PEOPLE

The servant-leader recognizes the awesome responsibility to nurture the personal and professional growth of those we come in contact with.

10. BUILDING COMMUNITY

The building of community is nurtured in institutions, large and small. Every business has a culture, almost always top -down. We profess the willingness to get involved.

Leadership to the Patient

You and your patients share the expectation of high level performance. By continuously employing the ethical and virtuous principles in a caring and compassionate way, a practitioner "walks the talk" in demonstrating the principles of professionalism.

Since patients inherently see us as leaders because of our power position, it is best to early on accept a leadership attitude with gratitude and humility.

Leadership to the Profession

Professions expect their members to work in a manner that upholds the integrity of colleagues, advance the scholarly foundations of research and academia, and promote good order and governance in regulating the profession. The opportunities for demonstrating leadership come in small, medium and large doses.

Volunteering for committee work with the regulator or professional association, assisting in local affairs of the profession, participating in clinical trials, and making oneself available for larger commitments to further the good of the profession, all contribute.

The simplest way to demonstrate leadership to one's colleagues is to connect and engage. Be active in your professional association and pursue continuing education. Post graduate education upholds our professing to maintain clinical competence; an integral part in protecting the public and part of the Social Contract's deal.

Leadership In The Community

The opportunities for serving one's community are varied and readily available. Professionals choose to get involved in activities which are directly related to one's knowledge, training and experience. Others volunteer in so-called "lay" activities.

Service clubs are organizations of community minded individuals, whose purpose is in gathering to improve the quality of life where they live and work. Service clubs feature fund raising projects, with money donated to worthy groups and individuals. Rotary, Lions, and Chambers of Commerce are just a few examples. Newly graduated practitioners derive benefit from networking with other like minded business people in their community.

Civic volunteering includes sitting on hospital boards and municipal health and wellness committees and using one's expertise to influence public policy.

Other good venues for demonstrating community leadership include little league sports organizations, arts, cultural clubs and church commitments. Society expects professionals to participate in these kinds of community leadership activities. The benefit to the professional provides some balance in one's personal life, providing a sense of community, and opportunities to meet future patients.

Responsibility to the Regulator

Practicing as a health care professional is a privilege, not a right. A license to practice is granted by a regulator under a legislative mandate. Practitioners must demonstrate competencies in order to practice their craft. (Regulatory bodies are known as Licensing Boards in the United States, Colleges in Canada and Councils in the UK.) Some professions operate as a collective of multiple regulators sharing functions with more than one group in the mix, all working collaboratively.

While all regulators share the same primary purpose, protection of the public, boards, colleges and councils have multiple functions; all subsumed under this primary role of public safety. This is a key part of the Social Contract's deal; society giving significant powers to professionals, with the promise that the professions will be accountable and will protect the public from practitioner misconduct.

Like any organization or business, regulators require an office, staff and money to operate. State and provincial laws require practitioners to submit to their regulator's authority and to declare annually a promise to practice within their scope of practice, are fit to practice, and declare they have not been involved in criminal activity or other civil misconduct.

While professionals enjoy a good degree of autonomy in choosing where to practice, there are limits. Licensure in one jurisdiction does not automatically allow a practitioner to move to another without being vetted. Applicants must submit their educational and work history, disclosing any impairments to their fitness to practice. Previous misconduct is to be disclosed so that the new jurisdiction can determine how effectively this has been addressed by the applicant.

Regulators have a duty to report on the activities of the profession to their own members, to government administrators and to the public. The public record forms a key part of a profession's commitment to public safety and protection.

Beyond annual relicensure, practitioners have a professional responsibility to be current with all published guidelines, statutes and standards of practice. While these proscriptions are set out and enforced by the regulator, it is the collective profession itself that creates them. In other words, a practitioner who believes they know better than a published standard of practice is in direct opposition to his or her peers.

Guidelines, statutes and standards of practice are wide ranging and cover much of a practitioner's work. Because they evolve over time, there is an ongoing responsibility to keep current. Full compliance with standards of practice is non-negotiable. Failure to comply gives rise to complaints. Patients and their family members, office staff, other professional colleagues, employers and insurers are common sources of complaint.

Regulatory governing bodies set out standards of practice and protocols which serve the public good. Codes of conduct and standards of behaviors set the minimum acceptable standards required by professional members. They might also be known as the "floor", delineating the line not to be transgressed.

While ideal behaviors and standards are not readily codified by law, it is the principles of professionalism that motivates a practitioner to aspire to the "ceiling."

Practitioner Discipline

Managing complaints is one important function of licensing bodies and part of the deal with society. While there are differences between jurisdictions and also between professions in the same locale, the usual sequence of events unfolds as follows:

- Receipt of the Complaint
  - Regulators require these to be issued, usually in writing though some permit electronic submissions.
- Notification
  - The practitioner is notified of the complaint and asked to respond.
  - Complainants are provided with the practitioner's response.
- Regulator Review
  - Submissions and responses are reviewed by a complaints committee comprised of peers and public members.
- Investigation
  - The complaints committee decides whether to launch a formal investigation.
- Decision
  - In due time the complaints committee will decide:
    - No further action (No Public Record)
    - Reminder (No Public Record)
    - Advice (No Public Record)
    - Caution (Public Record)
    - Remediation (Public Record)
    - Referral to Discipline (Public Record)
- Discipline Hearings
  - Matters for formal discipline may be tried by a separate discipline committee. This committee renders a decision and issues a penalty, based on the findings.
  - Appeals processes vary between jurisdictions

Scenarios and Searches

a. Search your regulator's website for past disciplinary decisions. What themes emerge? Apart from sexual and financial abuse, what other types of misconduct are reported? Note there are "public members" who are active in committee work on boards, colleges and councils. What specific responsibilities do these important non-practitioner public members have?

b. What does "Duty to Report" consist of with your regulator? What events or scenarios are you legally required to report?

c. Moral agency can be a difficult concept to grasp. It is predicated on both ethical and moral discernment, and power. The phrase "speaking truth to power" is often used in whistle-blowing situations. Explore what scenarios might fulfill a practitioner's duty to act as a moral agent. Drill deeper. On a personal level what issues strike you as being less than just in health care?

d. Explore the power of the professional's signature. When young, what time and effort did you put into perfecting the look you wanted in your signature? Why did this matter? Be current. What power comes with the practitioner's signature? By virtue of your professional authority, what are you able to do (or soon able to do) by signing a document? List those. What concerns are there with use of a stamped or electronic signature?

You be the judge

A surgeon was investigated for conducting a Facetime chat with another surgeon while still in the operating theatre. The conversation was personal; not clinical. One of the nurses reported this incident. The patient was anesthetized and the Facetime conversation occurred as the team finished up.

The incident was investigated by the hospital and the surgeon's defence was: (a) an experienced resident was tasked with completing the final steps; (b) there were no complications; (c) there was no privacy breach; and (d) the call lasted only 4 minutes.

If you were on the hospital discipline committee, would this constitute professional misconduct and possible referral to the regulator?

Further References and Resources

One chiropractic college dean denotes leadership as "the most crucial element missing in the profession." Any search on professional leadership reveals a paucity of peer reviewed citations. Don't shy away from the grey literature.

Brett, A.S., "Physicians have a responsibility to meet the health care needs of society," *Journal of Law, Medicine and Ethics,* 2012.

Brown, R.C.H., Savulescu, J., "Responsibility in healthcare across time and agents," *Journal of Medical Ethics,* 2019.

Lo, B., *Resolving Ethical Dilemmas; a guide for physicians,* 6th ed., Wolters Kluwer, 2019.

Gersh, M.R., "Servant-Leadership: a philosophical foundation in physical therapy," *Journal of Physical Therapy Education,* 2006.

McCullough, L.B., "An ethical framework for the responsible leadership of accountable care organizations," *American Journal of Medical Quality,* 2012.

Steering Committee on Modernization of Health Profession Regulation, Ministry of Health, British Columbia, *Recommendations to modernize the provincial health profession regulatory framework,* 2020.

CHAPTER 6

Fit to Practice

Caregivers well know the challenges of committing themselves to the rigors of patient care while constantly striving to maintain their own personal health and wellbeing. Call this a never-ending pursuit and an unavoidable dilemma. Despite this tension, the best caregivers "walk the talk" in modeling optimal health and wellness.

Regulators and educators concur that management of one's physical and mental health is a significant ethical issue, due to the potential harm to patients when a practitioner is less than fit.

Patients need their caregiver to be well. A healthy practitioner is an inspiring and affirming influencer. This is not idle opinion. Hippocrates proscribed such for his students: "Physicians should look healthy and as plump as nature intended; for the common crowd consider those who are not of this excellent bodily condition to be unable to take care of others." Turn the clock ahead a few thousand years and nothing needs to be changed; maybe not even the plump part!

Practitioners are reminded daily that health is not simply the absence of pain. The World Health Organization defines health as a state of optimal physical, mental and social well-being; not merely the absence of disease and infirmity. Caregivers use their fiduciary lens to advocate for this optimal state of healthy living in every patient seen.

The sad irony is that health care professionals easily become overwhelmed in work chores and face a constant struggle to find their own physical, mental and social well-being. Finding and then maintaining balance is difficult. Long before global pandemics took center stage, overwork, stress, burnout, relationship difficulties and dependence were shared experiences in health care communities. The *sequalae* affect our patients, our families and our colleagues.

A healthy professional is one that has achieved balance. Beyond the ability to deliver excellent clinical care, balance includes a cooperative and interdependent relationship with colleagues and staff, stable relationships with spouse and children, physical wellness, social interests removed from daily work and the ability to enjoy feelings of contentment and gratitude. This never happens by luck or chance, but reflection, design and proactive effort.

Balance and Objectivity

Balance is the ability to function well in multiple roles: caregiver, colleague, supervisor, spouse, parent, friend, volunteer; and maintain this high level of function while being healthy in body, mind and spirit.

Objectivity is the ability to discern whether sought after values, goals and objectives have been met; and knowing how to take action to meet these objectives. Objective insight refocuses our values to strategize with purpose and action. Stress, burnout, relationship struggles, impairment and addiction all threaten balance and objectivity.

Family Matters

To paraphrase Jesus' words in St. Matthew's gospel, what does it benefit a professional who accumulates patients, money and great accolades, but loses family members along the journey? The temptation to immerse ourselves in work to the detriment of our home duties and responsibilities never ends. Without discernment, balance and maintaining our own boundaries, we risk withdrawing from those who are closest to us, and investing our resources in temporal things which produce little inner peace and contentment.

Children grow up quickly. Practitioners have a key parental responsibility to carve out contact time with their kids. Quality time is not readily compartmentalized into a schedule. Objectivity, resolve and balance are the only remedies.

Competence

The Social Contract mandates that the professions are responsible in ensuring their members are safe and efficacious.

At the individual level there is a never-ending responsibility for a licensed practitioner to maintain competence. Every senior student knows the stress of board exams. Learners express few fears greater than completing all of their scholastic competencies, only to be denied the opportunity to practice because of a missed board exam.

Standards of practice are set by those who have gone before and are intended to uphold a high level of knowledge and skill. This rigor assures patients and the public of protection. Because the pace of change in health care requires practitioners to maintain competence, jurisdictions mandate continuing education as part of licensure.

The information age provides more stressors. As life-long-learners we now have the ready availability of evidence at our fingertips. The down side is the overwhelming amount of information needing assimilation in a finite amount of time. Woe to the busy-ness of an overloaded schedule and an unbalanced personal life; this being one formula leading to practitioner vulnerability. Such vulnerability while under-resourced is a precursor for errors in judgement. A forensic "looking back" sees this as the setting where egregious boundary violations may occur.

Civility

One measure of our fitness to practice is how we interact with those around us. Civility is defined as a professional competency in working well with others to achieve shared goals. It encompasses all aspects of team play and speaks to positive social interactions and respect for other team members.

Dr. Michael Kaufmann, architect of the Practitioner Assistance Program posits five fundamentals of civility:

- Treat everyone in the workplace with respect
- Be deliberate, mindful and aware of your actions
- Communicate effectively
- Model good self-care, health and wellness
- Take responsibility and accept personal accountability

An unwell, unfit practitioner is a hazard to workplace harmony and productivity. Any form of toxicity in the work environment harms colleagues and affects patient care.

Burnout

Burnout, a career adversity syndrome, is ubiquitous in health care.

Early signs of distress are irritability and mood swings. Burnout is characterized by exhaustion, depersonalization and a decreased sense of accomplishment and satisfaction. Physical symptoms are those seen in patients: headaches, gastrointestinal distress, muscle and joint aches, insomnia, fatigue, anhedonia and anorexia.

Emotional manifestations include cynicism, unresolved anger, negativity, withdrawal, feelings of hopelessness and disillusionment. Mental and spiritual signs include depression, anxiety, substance use and a loss of purpose. Social or family conflict and withdrawal occur early on so that spouses and children are the first to know something is wrong.

Demands from patients are met with the feeling of having nothing left to give. Cognitive difficulties affecting concentration, memory and problem solving are late-stage markers.

Impairment and Addiction

An impaired practitioner is one who is unable to practice with reasonable skill and safety because of a physical or mental illness. While impairment may be attributed to age related cognitive decline, more commonly regulators deal with practitioner substance abuse. Dependence and addiction are the inability to control use of alcohol or other drugs, and include preoccupation with using, physiological tolerance and withdrawal symptoms on cessation. Continued use leads to dependence.

An impaired practitioner poses great risk of harm to patients and has an elevated risk for severe personal health consequences including suicide.

Employee Assistance

While many practitioners perform their work as independent contractors and are self-employed, others are hired via a health care corporation or hospital contract. Employee Assistance Programs (EAP) provide support as part of worker entitlements.

An Employee Assistance Program focuses on one's psychological state, emphasizing the importance of a healthier, more productive person, at work and home.

These programs use a counsellor or psychotherapist to sort out personal difficulties including work-related stress, marital problems and dependence on alcohol and other drugs. The emphasis on short-term therapy focuses on clarifying the problem, implementing solutions and monitoring progress.

The key is the practitioner knowing when they need help. Self-awareness is a strategic virtue. Because workplaces ensure anonymity, employees are encouraged to seek help.

Reality Check

Not convinced at how relevant practitioner health and wellness is?

Published data have reported that each and every day in the United States of America at least one physician dies by suicide. This loss is incomprehensible. Governments at every level would take immediate action if, for example, a large jet filled with skilled professionals crashed periodically. We would take whatever steps necessary to ensure such a catastrophic event never occured again.

Getting Help

While practitioners go to great lengths to conceal their behaviors from work colleagues even when they are unable to disguise their problems at home, colleagues and staff are aware that one of their own is struggling. Caring individuals offer help.

Offers of help are met with denial. When confronted with irrefutable evidence of use or dependence, colleagues and family members often rely on the assistance of an outside party such as a rehabilitation service. Confronting and convincing a practitioner can be more readily facilitated with the practitioner being made aware that refusal will involve their regulator. Many jurisdictions use the practitioner assistance program for this very situation. Addicted practitioners are deserving of care, not punishment.

In those rare cases of self-awareness, primary care providers refer to treatment facilities for assessment and care. Some drug and alcohol rehabilitation facilities specialize in treatment of the health care practitioner. Self-care is never an option.

More Resources

Mental health resources come in different packages. Self-help groups include 12-step programs such as Alcoholics Anonymous, Narcotics Anonymous and Al-Anon (for co-dependents) found in all communities. Local municipalities have mental health resources available on referral from primary care physicians; some with specialized drug and alcohol treatment facilities. Clinical psychotherapy comes from different training backgrounds including psychology, psychiatry, social work and pastoral counseling. Treatment works.

It is erroneous to think one should wait until they hit their "bottom" to get help. The recommended first step is to talk to a trusted colleague, also known as "objective other." None of us are invincible. Asking for help is a sign of fortitude and discernment and walks the talk of professing.

Vacation's Value

There is a growing body of evidence that by taking regular vacations from work, a practitioner is able to maintain better physical and mental health. This lesson is a good one for every health professional and goes to the very core of who we are as humans. We all need rest from work.

Evidence shows that an increased frequency of vacations is directly related to a reduced rate of death from all causes including heart attack and stroke, a reduced tendency to depression and a higher quality of life. Health care practitioners see this in others routinely. Why would we not expect this to apply to us?

Humility

More than a century ago, when the modern era of medicine was emerging, Sir William Osler addressed his students: "Take the reed of humility in your hands. Appreciate the length of the way, the difficulties to overcome and the fallibility of your faculties."

Scholar Coulehan, provides a contemporary understanding of humility in health care with three qualities:

- Unflinching self-awareness
- Empathic openness to others
- A keen appreciation of, and gratitude for, the privilege of caring for others.

To be humble means having a modest or low view of one's importance. If a practitioner's primary goal is personal profit and prestige, there is no commitment to the primary goals of a profession: prevention, healing and palliation.

Your Professional Association

There are key differences between your licensing body, the regulator, and the professional association. While separate and distinct, learners confuse their roles. If the primary role of the regulator is protection of the public, what is the purpose of your profession's association?

Professional associations, also known as societies, are groups that advocate for the interests of the profession and its members. It is easy to be confused with the messaging professional associations disseminate. Rather than say something akin to "we're here for ourselves" official communication is always oriented to the public good.

Professional associations provide essential influence over the affairs of the profession and only in rare circumstances, directly oppose a licensing body. They provide necessary oversight to many aspects of organization, research, qualification and continuing education.

The notable contrast with the regulator is in granting licensure and undertaking professional discipline; these the exclusive functions of the licensing body. While a professional association may censure and expel members for conduct unbecoming to the profession, it does not have the legislated authority to suspend or revoke a member's license. It is easy to be confused as the public messaging from both entities professes protection of the public as the primary role with extolling the value of practitioners' care.

Associations rely on individuals to volunteer for committee work. They further rely on an active and robust membership to better further the shared goals of the profession. Young practitioners do well in finding such a niche to give back to the profession, fulfilling one's professing to "honor and uphold the profession."

Scenarios and Searches

a. Stress and burnout are ubiquitous. Download the Connor-Davidson Resilience Scale or a similar survey. Rate your stress management and resilience quotient at this current stage of your career.

b. Anticipate observing some form of unprofessional behavior with a colleague. It happens. What is a preferred way to handle concerns about a health care professional who appears to be unwell and may be putting patients and co-workers in harm's way?

c. Search for Dr. Michael Kaufmann's five defining aspects of "civility in health care." After reading each description and with personal reflection, identify which ones are your best, and least fulfilled ones.

d. Sooner or later you will be called on to care for a patient with celebrity status. Categories include politics, the arts, music or someone well known in the corporate world. Speak with a senior practitioner to understand the power dynamics at play when caring for a celebrity patient and what responsibilities the practitioner has to ensure care is delivered consistently and with high quality, and options for dealing with non-compliance.

You be the judge

A dentist was charged with DUI (impaired driving) late one Saturday night, having been found by police in a quiet residential neighborhood. He had pulled over to the side of the road and was slumped over in the driver's seat, with the engine still running. Two days later he attended the local police station and was told the DUI charge was officially dropped. He never told his office staff, nor patients nor anyone about the incident.

Six months later he received notice from his licensing council informing him that he was under investigation for an incident involving the police. He hired a lawyer and provided a statement to his licensing body saying there was no need to inform the regulator as the charge was reversed hours later, there was never a conviction, and he never heard from the police again.

You be the judge. Was this dentist guilty of "failure to report"?

Further References and Resources

It's tempting to prioritize some professionalism ideals over others. While we are allowed favorites, self-awareness is virtuous, though most of us need an objective "other" to sharpen our awareness.

Connell, G., Bainbridge, L., "Understanding how chiropractors build trust with patients: a mixed-methods study," *Journal of the Canadian Chiropractic Association,* 2020.

De Hert, S., "Burnout in healthcare workers: prevalence, impact and preventative strategies," *Local and Regional Anesthesia,* 2020.

Epstein, R.M., Krasner, M.S., "Physician resilience: what it means, why it matters, and how to promote it," *Academic Medicine,* 2013.

Iflaifel, M., Lim, R.H., Ryan, K. *et al.*, "Resilient health care: a systematic review of conceptualisations, study methods and factors that develop resilience," *BMC Health Services Research,* 2020.

Khan, A., Vinson, A.E., "Physician well-being in practice," *Anesthesia & Analgesia,* 2020.

McClafferty, H., Brown, O.W., "Physician health and wellness," *Pediatrics,* 2014.

Robertson, H.D., Elliott, A.M., Burton, C. *et al.*, "Resilience of primary healthcare professionals: a systematic review," *British Journal of General Practice,* 2016.

Wald, H.S., "Optimizing resilience and wellbeing for healthcare professions trainees and healthcare professionals during public health crises – practical tips for an 'integrative resilience' approach," *Medical Teacher,* 2020.

Yester, M., "Work-life balance, burnout, and physician wellness," *Journal of Health Care Management,* 2019.

You Be the Judge

The scenarios presented in this text are a composite of various health care practitioners' disciplinary outcomes. Professions and scenario details have intentionally been altered to obscure any identifying features, even though all details have been taken from public records.

Regulatory licensing bodies in every jurisdiction share one non-negotiable proscription: it is absolutely forbidden for a health care professional to enter into a concurrent treating and romantic/sexual relationship with a patient.

Other types and lesser severities of misconduct are subject to some relativity. Disciplinary panels consider all aspects of the practitioner's behavior and the real and potential harmful outcomes that have affected other parties. Penalties are commensurate with the severity of the misconduct.

Temporary suspension from practice allows for a focused period of reflection and appropriate remediation. Permanent revocation of a practitioner's license is very rare. Depriving patients and society of a skilled practitioner's expertise is the last step to be considered, and is only reserved for chronic re-offenders and those guilty of egregious sexual abuse.

If you disagree with the verdicts and penalties reported here, bear in mind some details and deliberations of disciplinary panels are not put on the public record, nor are any personal mitigating circumstances, such as mental health diagnoses. While these are not overlooked and often are part of an agreed statement of facts or consent orders, selected details may be protected.

You Be the Judge Verdicts

CHAPTER 1

The chiropractor's history taking was found acceptable. The examination protocols pointed to a list of differential diagnoses. Pulmonary embolism was not on the list. While the working diagnosis was incorrect, there was no indication that this constituted clinical negligence as an embolic event is extremely rare in an otherwise young and healthy patient.

However, the chiropractor was found guilty of misconduct in editing the patient's chart. Making edits and additional details after an encounter is permissible *provided the subsequent date is clearly noted.* The investigative committee concluded that "query pulmonary embolism" was made to look like it was part of the original differential list. Because this was not charted on the first visit, it gave the appearance of a cover-up; this constituting one form of misrepresentation. The practitioner was given a formal caution.

CHAPTER 2

There was no dispute from any party that the financial fraud was entirely that of the massage therapist. The physical therapist, the owner, had been fully cooperative with the insurance provider and the regulatory investigators.

The committee concluded that, while the massage therapist was completely at fault for the fraudulent billings, the physical therapist *was guilty of supervisory neglect.* Because the PT was the clinic owner and had assembled the caregiving team, the licensing body asserted that all billings sent by the clinic's practitioners were under the auspices and responsibility of the owner. No oversight check and balance provisions had been established for the clinic, but *should have been.* The owner was found guilty of supervisory neglect and required to take additional training in ethics and jurisprudence.

CHAPTER 3

A lengthy and detailed investigation examined every aspect of the practitioner's interactions with the patient; before and after her discharge.

- While there was no evidence there had been substandard in-patient care, the practitioner was found guilty of repeated boundary violations while she was hospitalized. He should not have shared intimate details of his personal life.
- Providing an in-patient with the caregiver's mobile number constituted a boundary violation.
- He had not waited a long enough period of time before entering into a friendship or romantic relationship and, should not have invited her to move into his residence.
- The practitioner was naïve to the power differential he had with patients and quite unaware of this patient's vulnerability.
- Sexual activity with a former patient was entirely self-gratifying without benefit to the former patient.
- The practitioner's conduct constituted sexual abuse and brought the reputation of the profession into disrepute.

The psychotherapist was found guilty of professional misconduct. His penalty included a 6 month license suspension and two courses of ethics remediation focusing on boundary setting and maintenance. The hospital terminated him with cause.

CHAPTER 4

The licensing body's investigation confirmed the veracity of the other party's allegations and considered two issues: was the other party a patient; and, does online sexual activity constitute a violation of the profession's moral standards?

- The other party was not a patient. There was no evidence that this relationship had anything to do with health or health care. No clinical advice or recommendations had been communicated. The practitioner was not guilty of a concurrent treating and sexual relationship.

- The second concern concluded the health care professional brought the entire profession into disrepute by engaging in gratuitous sexual activity with another party, even if online and anonymous. This was described as "moral turpitude." The licensing body asserted that regulated members are held to higher standards than the general public, and have a duty to uphold the high moral and ethical standards that society expects.

- The regulator asserted it *does* take an interest in practitioner conduct when not treating patients. This is to ensure that conduct outside of the office does not result in any effect on a practitioner's fitness to practice, in addition to behavior that might tarnish the reputation of the profession.

CHAPTER 5

One of the surgical nurses filed an official complaint with the hospital administrator. A small investigative team interviewed all those who had been working on this surgical event, though the surgeon refused to provide the name of the other party, to the investigators.

- The committee concluded that the surgeon had a duty of care to the others in the surgical suite: patient, resident, nurses and the hospital itself.

- Despite the brevity of the Facetime call, there was no legitimate reason to be removed from the completion tasks at hand.
- The surgeon was found guilty of professional misconduct and ordered to take training in ethics and professionalism. The surgeon had a fiduciary duty to the other parties and should have been fully and actively engaged in completing the procedure before anything else.
- The hospital stated that non-compliance or any future recurrence would result in referral to the licensing body.

CHAPTER 6

The licensing board was informed of the criminal charge by the police sargeant who had been assisting the arresting officer. This information was reported to the board two weeks after the charge was dropped. An investigation revealed that the dentist had prior history with the board. Six years before this event, a hygienist had alleged the dentist had often been late for work, often appearing to be hung over. At that time there was no specific misconduct identified but the dentist was referred to the Practitioner Assistance Program in order to be assessed for possible drug or alcohol dependence.

The dentist was found guilty of failure to report. The licensing body stipulated that any member who had been charged criminally was duty-bound to inform the regulator within 30 days, *even if charges were stayed or dropped.* It mattered not whether the criminal charges were laid during the practitioner's work activities or when not involved in patient care.

Failure to report constituted professional misconduct. The dentist was ordered to undergo a second assessment with the PAP and take additional training in ethics and jurisprudence.

www.ingramcontent.com/pod-product-compliance
Lightning Source LLC
Chambersburg PA
CBHW040901210326
41597CB00029B/4928